Autobiographies
of **Our Orgasms**

A Collection of Your Stories
VOLUME TWO

Edited by Betsy Blankenbaker

CONTENTS

DEDICATION III

FOREWORD V

NOTE TO READERS: VII

ONE 9
THE NEW WOMEN'S LIB:
FREE YOUR ORGASM
BY BETSY BLANKENBAKER

TWO 15
YEAR OF THE YONI
BY MANDY NOLAN

THREE 21
A RESURRECTION
BY GLORIA JANE

FOUR 29
IT'S ALL IN YOUR HEAD
BY ESME STARK

FIVE 37
CONNECTING THE DOTS
BY TRACEY ALLRED

SIX 49
I LOVE MY LADYSCAPE
BY LISA LISTER

SEVEN 55
PUPPIES AND PUSSIES
BY JANE MILLER

EIGHT 59
HEALING THE HEALER
BY ROBYN DALZEN

NINE 71
THE BOX
BY KIM SHIRLEY

TEN 77
**BEYOND THE CLASSROOM
AND INTO THE CURRICULUM OF ORGASM**
BY DR. E. POWELL

ELEVEN 89
REMEMBERING WHO I AM
BY M.R. GONZALEZ

TWELVE 97
RECLAMATION OF MY ORGASM
BY CINDY ANNE

THIRTEEN 103
THIS WILD RISE
BY REBECCA HOLT

FOURTEEN 135
50 SHADED POEMS
BY CASSY FRY

FIFTEEN 139
SEXUALITY AT ITS PEAK
BY LEIGH HURST

SIXTEEN 151
FIRE IN MY PUSSY
BY DEBORAH PENNER

SEVENTEEN 161
HOW TO TURN ME ON
BY MARY JAMES

EIGHTEEN 169
**WHAT MY ORGASM WANTS
TO TELL YOU**
BY BETSY BLANKENBAKER

ACKNOWLEDGEMENTS 171

DEDICATION

For each person who wrote to me after reading *Autobiography of an Orgasm* but is still too afraid to speak up – these stories are for you.

FOREWORD

From the moment I read Betsy's first book, **Autobiography of an Orgasm**, I was impressed with how important and essential her words were for me, my patients, and for women everywhere. Revealing the truths of our bodies creates a necessary path to breaking the cycle of silence and awakening the life force and powerful healer that resides in each of us - our orgasm. Her books, real stories from real women, show us the way. I knew upon meeting her that she and I were on a similar mission to help make the womb a healthier place.

Dr. Liz Orchard
Naturopathic Medical Doctor
Founder of Be Well Natural Medicine Clinic
www.bewellnaturalmedicine.com

NOTE TO READERS:

This work is memoir. It reflects each writer's present recollection of his or her life. In some stories, certain names, locations, and identifying characteristics have been changed. Dialogue and events have been recreated from memory to convey the substance of what happened, and they represent each writer's recollection of the events. Several writers chose to publish under a pseudonym for privacy.

The use of American or UK spelling and punctuation standards vary depending on the writer.

ONE

THE NEW WOMEN'S LIB: FREE YOUR ORGASM

by Betsy Blankenbaker

In 1963, the year I was born, The Feminine Mystique was published. The author, Betty Friedan, made the case that women needed to "find" themselves, that women longed for an identity beyond the tradition role of "sexual passivity, male domination and nurturing maternal love" that was a common experience for women at the time. Freidan wrote, "Our culture does not permit women to accept or gratify their basic need to grow and fulfill their potentialities as human beings, a need which is not solely defined by their sexual role."

After the book's release, the seeds were planted for the Women's Liberation movement, and women of the 1960s and 70s demanded social, political and economic freedom.

The liberation didn't end there. There was also a sexual revolution that led to the publishing of the book *Our Bodies, Ourselves* in 1971. Until then, most women received information about their bodies only from their doctors, who were predominately male. The book, which sold four million copies, offered women information about their bodies, health and

9

sexuality. It was a call for women to take full ownership of their bodies. It was liberating, but it was not enough.

It's been fifty years since the beginning of the Women's Liberation movement. Today women have access to more information than ever about their bodies and sex. Why then, with all this advancement, are we still accepting that one in five of us has sexual dysfunction? Where is the liberation?

For many years, I was the one in five.

In her book *Vagina*, Naomi Wolf writes, "Female sexual pleasure, rightly understood, is not just about sexuality or just about pleasure. It serves, also, as a medium of female self-knowledge and hopefulness; female creativity and courage; female focus and initiative; female bliss and transcendence; and as a medium of sensibility that feels very much like freedom. To understand the vagina properly is to realize that it is not only coextensive with the female brain, but it is also, essentially, part of the female soul."

I spent five years researching orgasm as a way to understand my body and its ability to feel ecstasy after a lifetime of feeling nothing. It's those inside wounds that we can't heal with Band-Aids, so they stay with us for years until we either die with them or we finally sit with them, like I did when I wondered at the age of forty-five why I had a life that looked good but didn't feel good.

I ignored my orgasm for years. It helped me ignore the trauma my vagina experienced when I was molested by a neighbor as a child and assaulted as a teenager. I ignored my orgasm through an abortion in college. I ignored my orgasm through two marriages and five births. I ignored my orgasm when I was raped at the age of forty. I ignored my orgasm because I didn't think I deserved to feel good after so much damage. I was the one in five disconnected from my body. I was the one in five disconnected from my soul.

The medical industry diagnoses us with female sexual dysfunction. One common "solution" is to prescribe an anti-depressant. I was offered Prozac. Did my doctor think I was depressed or did he think my vagina was depressed?

If one in five women are diagnosed with female sexual dysfunction and one in three women experience assault against their bodies in their lifetime, maybe our vaginas are shutting down from either the abuse or from accepting that "it's hard for women to orgasm" because that's the message we hear over and over again.

I spent years going to doctors who told me what was wrong with me until finally I started to look to myself to find what was right with me. It occurred to me that women, including myself, had been given a lot of misinformation about our bodies and orgasm. My healing finally came through the one thing I'd been avoiding all those years—I liberated my orgasm.

I started researching my body and its ability to feel, as if I were an anthropologist on a sacred exploration for the truth. I read books and took courses and workshops in sexuality and sensuality, but the real learning came from listening to my own body's wisdom. I wanted to become the sexual authority on my body, and along the way I also became the spiritual authority, too. My body became my preacher.

With practice, I was surprised how quickly my being came back to life as I allowed myself to feel my orgasm. I committed to training my body in the same way that Michael Jordan practiced basketball or Einstein committed to science.

"We should be teaching our daughters and granddaughters to familiarize themselves with their anatomy and let them know that many girls and women explore and touch their genitals for the sake of pleasure," writes Dr. Christiane Northrup in *Goddesses Never Age*.

One of the biggest shifts for me was understanding the difference between orgasm and climax. It's not difficult for a woman to orgasm when you understand that it begins with the first sensation you feel when your body is turned on. The butterflies in your belly. The tingling of your inner thighs. The flood of warmth in your genitals. That is part of your orgasm. Your climax is when your body takes you over the top edge of your orgasm and then the sensations slow down and stop. But your orgasm, all those feelings, can be sustained as long as you stay present, following the good sensations with or without a climax.

11

There are eight thousand nerve endings in a woman's clitoris, solely dedicated to making her feel good. We were born with them, a gift from the Creator. Those nerve endings never go away, but if ignored, the pathways of energy that send doses of a feel-good hormone straight to our brains can't do their jobs, so we end up self-medicating with Prozac or alcohol, or we believe that it's hard for us to feel our orgasm and climax. It is not!

My friend Dr. Liz Orchard explained to me that "Revealing the truths of our bodies creates a necessary path to breaking the cycle of silence and awakening the life force and powerful healer that resides in each of us— our orgasm."

Research shows that orgasm and climax with a trusted, loving partner bring about the ultimate state of health for both people. I was mostly experiencing my orgasms and climaxing on my own through self-cultivation—a term I prefer over masturbation. Self-cultivation floods your body with feel-good chemicals. I was healing myself and I was nourishing myself. I was creating ultimate states of health through my orgasm. Various aches in my body and imbalances that I'd had for years disappeared. My skin glowed and my mood improved. When I looked in the mirror, I saw a different face—younger, more relaxed—even my eyes sparkled. Several friends asked if I'd had "work" done on my face. It was just my orgasm. Life started to feel good again.

Maybe our vaginas are not depressed. Maybe they're asking to be liberated from the sex we're sold through the media, through church, through porn, through the men in our lives who don't know any better because we haven't asked for it. Our culture rarely gives girls and women the message to honor their bodies as sacred. We wouldn't give ourselves away or fake it if we treated ourselves with reverence. Maybe we'll truly be liberated when we value our entire essence as women After all, only women are born with a clitoris whose only function is to make us feel good. Maybe freeing our orgasm—our soul—is the ultimate women's liberation.

About the Author
Betsy Blankenbaker
www.betsyblankenbaker.com

What did you want to be when you were eight years old?

I loved writing and reading when I was young. I watched my parents read the morning and evening papers every day, so I decided to publish a paper for the kids in my neighborhood (and I also sold it to the adults for 10 cents). I called it *Booze in the News*. I had no concept what booze meant at that age. I only knew it rhymed with "news" and I thought it was a catchy title. The paper had news, comics and an advice column, all content created by me. I still have a copy of one of the editions of *Booze in the News*.

If you could give advice to your younger self about your orgasm (or your body), what would it be?

The *Wizard of Oz* was a favorite movie of my childhood (and even now). When I was younger, I wished I really understood the bigger message of Glinda, the Good Witch, as she spoke these words to Dorothy: "You've always had the power, my dear. You've had it all along. "

If your orgasm had a voice, what would it say to you about the piece you wrote for this book?

You are part of a bigger movement to help women remember the power, healing and ultimate states of health and wellness that exist when we give our body (and life) permission to feel good.

Anything else?

I write about sexuality and the sacred body. My first book, *Autobiography of an Orgasm*, goes beyond the physical to the spiritual experiences of being a woman. I was born in Indiana—the conservative heartland of the United States—and raised my four children between Indiana and Miami. I now live as a nomad, making my home around the world as I teach. This book was written between "homes" in Bali, Australia and the U.S. Traveling so much in recent years made me think about home and my lack of feeling rooted. I now realize it may have something to do with abuse by a teenage neighbor within my childhood home and not feeling safe there. The gift of this has been to heal myself so I finally feel safe in my true home, my body.

Two

YEAR OF THE YONI

by Mandy Nolan

A few years ago I had a vagina. It was fairly common. All women I know had one. I was pretty happy with it; I think like most, mine was standard issue. It did the job nicely, thank you very much. I never really thought I needed the upgrade, but sometimes you don't get a say in it. Like a cosmic cootie coincidence, all at once we had our vaginas upgraded to the new improved more spiritual and endlessly more complex model: The Yoni. Who decided this should happen?

It's like I fell asleep with a regulation-issue vag and then suddenly woke up with some sort of spiritual vagina cave womb that now requires massage and worshipping and lots and lots of workshops to keep it happy. It seems to be very labour-intensive. From what I read in the *Echo* each week and spy on the web, I realise I could devote my entire work week to Yoni worship and still not touch the sides. Yep, it's all about the Yoni. In fact, when one looks at word usage over time, it's clear we are at peak Yoni. And in some cases, peaking Yoni (that's if you know the special 15-minute regulation yoni massage).

Yes, 2015 was the definitely the Year of the Yoni. Personally I think the good old-fashioned vagina was a lot easier to manage. It didn't require quite so much reverence, and it certainly didn't get its own special pants-off yoga class. Our sexual partners were much more at ease dealing with a vagina. While at times confusing, perplexing and with some startup problems, most had worked their way into a basic level of proficiency. Not so with the Yoni. Yoni work takes mastery. To operate a Yoni you need to be certified. It's like sitting on a temple. Shoes off at the front door of my Yoni, thank you very much. And by the way, Yonis don't do porn. Far too sacred for something as cheap and degrading as that. Yonis do sacred stuff like birthing babies, multiple orgasms and universe creation. I'm hoping we'll eventually find a Yoni that can solve the climate change riddle and reduce world hunger.

For those of you who don't know, *yoni* is a Sanskrit word that basically means to unite. I get that bit, being metaphoric and labial all at the same time, but it gets a bit weird when you really go deep. According to one definition, the yoni is the crucible where things are combined, where creation and re-creation takes place. Where the unseen world takes material form.' Wow, that is some multi-functioning device we girls have down there. No wonder it requires so much attention. And there I was, thinking its purpose was purely biological with a penchant for pleasure.

As an owner-operator of a vagina I will admit it's some impressive engineering—in fact, may I be so bold as to suggest that it's the original 3D printer? We girls have been printing small humans for years. On the Yoni. Don't even need ink cartridges. We are 100% organic people printers. While that's clearly worthy of a Nobel Prize or at the very least an episode on *Grand Designs* or *The New Inventors*, I have to say I didn't actually want a Yoni. I was more than happy with my very ordinary, non-sacred, easy-to-please vagina. You can do as many workshops as you want, but you will never please a woman with a Yoni. Not possible. We're talking one man (or woman) up against a force of universal creation. Talk about intimidating. It's like doing a spontaneous one-man show at the Sydney Opera House and hoping for a standing ovulation. So if we girls have the Yoni—what about the blokes?

Interestingly I don't see a lot of lingam worship workshops on offer. (*Lingam* is Sanskrit for the shaft of light, AKA the erect penis.) This lack of lingam could be due to the fact that the cock workshop has been going on for so long we no longer need to give the poor old Ganges worm a spiritual name, as 'cock' is pretty well dominant culture. That being said, after much careful consideration I have decided to not take up the offer of a Yoni and have sent it back. Instead I have stayed with the vagina. While it's not hands-free, it's much more user-friendly.

About the Author
Mandy Nolan
Mother of five, Mandy Nolan is a comedian and author
www.mandynolan.com.au

What I Would Do If I Were You
By Mandy Nolan
(available on Booktopia, Amazon, Kobo, iBooks)

A comedian's hilarious, sharply observed take on the bizarre events that make up day-to-day family life.

"Every morning I wake up and I think, Today, I am going to be a nice person. But I can't do it. By 8 o'clock I have lost my mind. Every day my kids act like the whole concept of getting up and going to school is a brand new idea. 'What, we're going to school? Really, what a surprise!' Of all the parenting routines, it's the morning routine that turns my head inside out"

Welcome to the wonderful, slightly wacky world of Mandy Nolan. She is a stand-up comedian, an artist, and a mother of five children ranging in age from grade school to university. Her on-stage accounts of everyday events of family life have entertained audiences for years. This hilarious collection of stories centered around Mandy's chaotic and slightly dysfunctional family life-and her attempts to be like the perfect, ideal mother she knows exists, somewhere. Mandy's perspective on home life and all its complications is delightfully unconventional and, above all, wickedly funny. Her humorous take on the bizarre events and mundanities of daily life are honestly and sharply observed—whether it is trying to revive her children's dying guinea pig, coping with their Facebook friends, explaining the dangers of sex and drugs (while hoping desperately they don't find out about her own past indiscretions), battling against head lice, or struggling to regain her own disappearing self-identity.

Boyfriends We've All Had (and Shouldn't Have)
By Mandy Nolan
(available on Booktopia, Amazon, Kobo, iBooks)

A raunchy laugh-a-minute romp through the dating mistakes we all make before finding Mr Just Right and settling down in the 'burbs. Written with Mandy's customary wit and punch, BOYFRIENDS is an entertaining read for Mother's Day. *In Boyfriends We've All Had (and Shouldn't Have)* Mandy Nolan turns her acerbic wit onto boyfriends past … and no one escapes her observations. From the needy, besotted drip to the brooding, unavailable bad boy, from Mr New Age to Mr Emotional Retard, Mandy has seen them all come and go in her quest for Mr Right. This is a hilarious and revealing look at the emotional, pot-boiling mess and angst of every type of romantic relationship.

Home Truths
By Mandy Nolan
(available on Booktopia, Amazon, Kobo, iBooks)

In *Home Truths*, comedian and author Mandy Nolan explores the significance of place in relationship to self, specifically what it is about home that is so intrinsic to our sense of self and what is says about our place in the world and our emotional, mental and spiritual wellbeing. This is a book about who we are in the place where we live, and why; it's about who we are when no-one is watching, when the doors are closed and the pants come off.

Mandy leaves no corner of our suburban psyches undisturbed in her clean-out of our comfort cobwebs, using her comedic talents to unearth insights buried behind closed doors, including:

o   Do shared houses unleash the hidden and very messy inner monster hiding within us all?
o   What does your rental property say about your approach to life?

o   What will the neighbours learn by perving through your windows or rummaging through the leftover detritus of past relationships that now grace your garage sale? and

o   Were people less troubled by obesity when their chairs and beds were more uncomfortable and pain forced them to get up earlier and rest less? Have plasma TVs and plush-cushioned comfort made us fat? It was on her knees unpacking the dishwasher that Nolan had one of her most important epiphanies.

'Life is not all about choice. Sometimes it's about subjugating one's own desires and ego at the service of the mundane. My daily rituals, my chores, the endless grind, this is the anvil that anchors my ego to the ground, that stops me floating skywards, becoming puffed up and unbearable...There are many people who would benefit from laundry therapy. I wonder when James Packer last washed his own undies?'

In *Home Truths*, Mandy explores the symptoms and the roots of this love of comfort, tracing our deluded nostalgia and the disappointment that is the result of going back to revisit the buildings and landmarks of our past. Everything seems so much smaller, more still and less impressive. Places that were magical in childhood are exposed as ordinary in adulthood.

THREE

A RESURRECTION

by Gloria Jane

An urgent knock on the door yanked me out of the romantic world of Jane Eyre and Edward Rochester and plopped me back in the reality of a dingy apartment in Little Rock, Arkansas. *Rude.* I silently placed my love-worn paperback on the coffee table and tiptoed over to the door, not wanting to let an unwelcome visitor know that I was home. I peered through the peep-hole… and I melted. It was *him*. It was Anthony, my lover. God, he was beautiful. I watched him for a moment, admiring his muscular body, visible through his snug t-shirt. I imagined removing the shirt, caressing his hard pecs underneath. Another, more insistent knock came, once again bringing me to reality. I opened the door, laughing to myself that this beautiful specimen of a male was mine, even if only for the summer.

"You've got to come with me. Right now," he said, and he took my hand. I hastily grabbed my keys and shut the door behind me. He didn't look anxious, exactly. He was excited. But we didn't head for his place; we headed for Wal-Mart.

"Wal-Mart?" I exclaimed. "Why on earth…?" But he wouldn't answer my questions. When we got there, he once again took me by the hand and briskly led me straight to the book section. I had read a stage play and a

21

screenplay he had written, both of which showed great potential, but he hadn't mentioned that he had published a book. When we got to the Harlequin Romance section, he paused and started skimming the shelves.

"Here." He pulled a book off the shelf, looked at it, held it to his chest, and took a big breath. Then he turned the book around for me to see. There he was. Not as author. No, he was the cover model on the front of a steamy romance novel, and he was perfect. I don't even recall if there was a woman in the picture. All I remember is him—his beautifully sculpted face, his strong arms that I had felt around me so many times in the past few weeks. *Him.* I looked up at him, his eyes betraying his fear that I would laugh at him, think him shallow. He was proud of this accomplishment and wanted to share it with me, even if he was too humble to just *tell* me. It was one of his many charms. I put my hand on his face, on that chiseled jawline that managed to have a five o'clock shadow at all times. I said, "It's beautiful. Thank you so much for sharing this moment with me." Then he took me home and showed me how much he appreciated me.

He wasn't my Edward Rochester. I knew that from the start. He was just a sexy man that I decided I wanted and somehow got for a while. When the inevitable end of our time together came, and he returned to his home in Los Angeles, I was sad but not heartbroken. He had been a passionate lover, one who was far more attentive to my needs than gorgeous men typically are. He was funny. He once bench-pressed me in bed, just to see if he could. (He could. And then he dropped me on his face, and we both laughed until we cried.) In the weeks after he left, as I finished reading *Jane Eyre* for the umpteenth time, I started wondering who my Edward was.

I was thirty-one years old. I had spent the past nine years of my life traveling for my job. I was ready for a change. I wanted to settle down in one place, with one man. Buy a house, start a family—you know, the American Dream. I started really thinking about the lessons I had learned that had brought me to this point in my life. I had been told that physical chemistry wasn't the most important thing in a lasting relationship. It was more important to be compatible emotionally, intellectually, spiritually, maybe even politically... but the chemistry sure felt good.

During my five-month stay in Little Rock, I met a lot of terrific people. I was a regular at all of the River Market bars and restaurants, and I soon had a close-knit circle of friends that I realized I would be happy to keep. One of these friends was a man named James. He was on the management team at a local bar, and he was awesome. We had a lot of similar interests, saw eye-to-eye on practically every topic... and unfortunately, I was not remotely physically attracted to him. We would sit for hours at a time, just talking and laughing and drinking. At the end of every conversation, he would remark that we had "great chemistry." I thought of Anthony. I knew what great chemistry was, and I certainly didn't have that with James. Don't get me wrong, I liked him a lot. I had a great deal of respect for him. He was really good at his job and at reading people.

He was also a divorcee. His ex-wife lived on the west coast with his nine year-old daughter. Never, in all of my daydreams about what my future husband would be like, did he have an ex-wife or children from a previous marriage. I was raised in a family where divorce simply didn't happen. But the more time I spent with him, the more I liked and respected him. And one week, while he was away visiting his daughter on the other side of the country, I realized that I missed him. *Really* missed him. My best friend happened to be in town visiting, and I told her about James. She just smiled at me, never one to tell me what to do. "What??" I insisted. But she just smiled.

I decided to give James a try. When he came back from California, I told him so. His response? "I knew you would come around." We started dating.

Our first kiss was disappointing, to say the least. He had big, squishy lips that didn't feel right against mine. *But he's an awesome guy, Gloria. He's a terrific friend.* So, I kept trying. Although the kissing (as well as other physical expressions of intimacy that I began to allow) never felt any better, I got used to them. I convinced myself that physical attraction was not that important. *Isn't that what you've come to learn in your thirty-plus years?*

You are looking for your second self, like Jane. You are looking for your equal. Isn't that why the universe brought James to you? Besides, all of our mutual friends thought we were the perfect match.

Many months later, after we had moved in together, I came home to find a ring box on the coffee table. There was a note that read, "Be my permanent chick." That was his proposal, and I accepted it. I know what you're thinking, dear reader. But please believe me when I say, it was truly the proposal I thought I wanted. I guess I am what you'd call a "closet romantic." I'm all tough on the outside. I don't need anyone. I don't like to be needed by anyone. That's what I let James see, and that's how he treated me in return.

We got married about two years after we met. It was a simple ceremony, and it was a ton of fun. But I was dreading the honeymoon. I couldn't admit that to myself at the time, but looking back and remembering the utter lack of lingerie that I packed, I was not looking to seduce my new husband. Not one bit.

Our sex life was dull and monotonous, and I didn't want to do anything to spice it up. I just wanted it *over with*. When we decided to start a family, we had more sex than ever. James was thrilled. I bore it. And much to my surprise, when I found out I was pregnant, he stopped wanting to have sex with me. *Yippee!! Can I spend our entire life pregnant, then?*

Having a baby ruined every single good thing about our marriage. We had to work opposite hours in order to take care of our precious little girl. We hardly ever saw each other. All of those hours we used to spend together just talking, laughing, and drinking? Those were a thing of the past. I returned to work when my daughter was three weeks old, which was an agonizing but necessary measure. James was left at home with a screaming child who wanted nothing to do with him. (She came by that honestly, huh?) I would receive heart-wrenching texts from him while in the middle of a meeting: "If she doesn't stop screaming, I'm going to throw her out the window." Of course he didn't actually *mean* those things, but I was stuck at work and couldn't offer any assistance. I began to resent him for even being willing to *have* a child with me if he couldn't handle the daily pressures of being a dad. He began to resent me for wanting a child in the first place. Literally, the only time James and I saw each other was during the "hand-off" where one of us would pass our child over to the other and mumble, "Good luck."

James began sleeping in the guest room. He would come into "my" room every other month or so for an obligatory romp in the hay, but either my obvious lack of desire for him or his increasing age and stress level began causing him problems in bed. He started having difficulties achieving and maintaining an erection. He went to a doctor and got a prescription to "help things." When I found out how much money he spent for an erection I didn't even *want*, well, that might have be the proverbial straw that broke our marriage all to hell.

He knew, of course, that I didn't want him. But one day, he made me say it out loud. It was not an easy conversation. I loved him dearly, and I still do, but more like a sibling than as a spouse. When I was finally able to put that into words, it crushed him. In my mind, this meant that we would just continue to live together as a family, but without the expectation of sex. In his mind, it meant divorce. He had no desire to share a home, a life, and a bed with me as an unwilling sexual partner.

In our first five years of marriage, not only did I not desire my husband, I didn't desire anyone. I didn't even have any desire to masturbate. I thought my libido was dead. Literally dead. The winter I turned thirty-nine, that all changed.

I happened to meet Chad. I don't know why, but I wanted him the moment I laid eyes on him, much like Anthony in Little Rock. None of my friends understood the attraction. He was not a Harlequin Romance cover model. He was a regular guy in a polo shirt and khakis. But it didn't matter, anyhow. I was happily married, right? I was still trying to convince myself I was. Well, this guy literally made me tongue-tied stupid. I couldn't be in the same room with him and breathe normally. It was *delicious...* and embarrassing! Well, his temporary position in my company ended, and I didn't see him again for another year. But let me tell you, this man haunted my dreams, day and night. I never stopped thinking about him, wanting him. He was my "material" when I had to have sex with my husband. I would squeeze my eyes shut and try to pretend that I was with Chad instead.

A year later, our paths crossed again. By that point in my life, my marriage was over, and James was moving out. I had never really expected to see Chad again, and the thrill of running into him was immediate and all-consuming. The time apart had done nothing to diminish my desire for him. I was just as tongue-tied stupid as I had been the year before. *Man, this guy must think I'm an idiot!* The weeks he spent with our company passed much as they had the year before, with me making a fool of myself repeatedly and Chad appearing not to notice. When his time with us drew to a close, I decided to make a move. (I'm not known for my impeccable timing.) But I was literally too ditzy around him to put an intelligible sentence together, so I sent him a text—just a simple, "I'll miss having you around" type of thing—and he texted back. He had been interested all along but wasn't sure where things stood in my personal life. And now he was leaving again.

What started as casual flirting via text soon progressed into something very intense. It was easier for me to be myself over the phone and through texts and emails, when his pheromones weren't so distracting. As we didn't live in the same city, it was months before we were able to see each other in person. When we finally set up a time to get together, my nerves were so frazzled I wasn't sure I'd be able to go through with it. But go through with it I did.

The first thing he did when I got to his house was to say, "You've been travelling. Why don't you shower?" Um, okay. When I got out, there was a luxurious white robe (like the kind you see in expensive hotels) waiting for me. I wrapped myself up in it, and he appeared with two glasses of red wine. He handed me one of them with a bit of a smirk. "Relax," he encouraged. I gratefully accepted and took a sip. It was perfect. Not too tannic, not too sweet. Then he took me by the hand and led me to his bedroom.

Our first kiss was tentative, but the second was electrifying. I could feel indescribable desire in every single cell of my body. I was positively humming with it. I could feel his excitement pressed firmly against me, and I thought I might just explode before my robe ever hit the floor. Then he slowly untied the belt…

Two hours and eight orgasms later (well, ten if you count his as well), I was collapsed on the floor, face down. He had collapsed on top of me. I might have even had a little rug-burn on my face. But I had never been more grateful in all of my life. I was grateful to all of the gods that humanity has ever worshipped. I was grateful for the gift of being a woman. I was grateful for every last nerve-ending, not just the ones in my clitoris. My *whole body* was singing. I was grateful for this re-awakening— not just of my libido and orgasm—but of my *self*, of my soul. I had spent so many years of my life telling me that physical attraction wasn't important. But I was no longer in denial.

It has been two and a half years since that memorable night. There have been many, many more memorable encounters with Chad. My sex life with him is beyond fulfilling. We don't see each other often, but we make our time together count. Two and a half years later, and I still tremble when he kisses me. My cells still ache for him. Do I ever fantasize that our relationship was something *more* than just sex? Occasionally. Do I ever wonder if I might love him, or if he might love me? Sometimes. Have I finally found my "Edward"? Nope. But in truth, this is all I need. I have a precious daughter whom I love, and who loves me, completely and unconditionally. I have a terrific circle of friends that I can rely upon. And I have a lover who I yearn for with every fiber of my being and who satisfies me completely. I'd say I'm a pretty lucky gal. Not Jane, just Gloria Jane.

About the Author
Gloria Jane
gloriajaneauthor@gmail.com

What did you want to be when you were eight years old?

I wanted to be a nurse.

If you could give advice to your younger self about your orgasm, what would it be?

I wouldn't! Every choice, every mistake, every good and bad thing that has ever happened to me has led me to be where I am right now... which is a pretty good place!

If your orgasm had a voice, what would it say to you about the piece you wrote for this book?

Glad you finally got this figured out!

Anything else?

Never settle. Don't just listen to your heart. Listen to your whole self.

FOUR

IT'S ALL IN YOUR HEAD

by Esme Stark

They say good sex is less a function of what goes on between our legs and more what happens between our ears. In my case, this proved true. Literally.

I was thirty-eight when it all went off the rails. My mother died one December afternoon as a result of a massive cerebral hemorrhage. Within the next few months, first one and then the other of my elderly dogs died. The company for which I worked—very contentedly—was acquired by another, and my job would be either made unbearable or eliminated altogether. And at home, my relationship was in critical condition. My partner was borderline bipolar, and when he was no longer getting the amount of attention he required, he behaved badly, often self-medicating with Glen Fiddich.

One of his grievances was that our sex life had deteriorated. My libido had gone missing. Well, you don't say, I thought. Do you think it might be stress-related? Or stemming from grief? Or that I sincerely suspect our relationship is on the rocks and don't trust you, which is compounding both the grief and the stress?

He badgered me to see a doctor to find a solution to what he termed my problem. This was a man who refused to see any professionals about his own vertiginous mood swings, because he was convinced they would prescribe drugs that might hog-tie his mind, which he perceived as brilliant, and others, including his supervisor, saw as simply manic. He seemed confident, however, that a doctor could give me a pill that would magically restore my libido.

To be fair, I resisted the notion of seeking medical advice almost as strenuously as he did. I could only imagine the eye-rolling that would follow my announcement that I'd come to ask where my sex drive might have gone. I could predict the flat, bored, professional stare, followed by any number of comments. *It's just a function of your age. It's only the stress; it will pass. Women don't have much libido – that's the way it is. Have you tried taking some vitamins?*

In the end, making a last-ditch effort to salvage my relationship played only a fractional part in my decision to make the appointment. I realized that the problem extended far beyond our bed—I no longer enjoyed any kind of physical activity. The happy feeling of well-worked muscles after a hike or an aerobics class was gone. My hairstylist's ministrations, all the shampooing, snipping and fussing, produced a lovely cut but no joy. My whole body seemed to have gone numb.

I had lost all interest in sex; my previously healthy appetite had vanished. I was purely incapable of reaching climax, either with him or on my own. One weekend morning when I had the house to myself, I headed off to the spare bedroom with a tube of lubricant and grim determination. I conjured up my most flammable fantasies as I stroked myself, yet my mind wandered off... Were there any green olives in the fridge? Did the lawn need mowing? In the past, I'd compared my climaxes to BASE-jumping off El Capitan. After what seemed like an hour of dogged effort, this one, barely perceptible, was more like stepping off a curb. Even the pleasure of touch, the delicious chill of fingers lightly stroking skin, was no more.

Hardest to explain was the experience of libido vacating my mind. I didn't feel the slightest frisson when I saw attractive men. I don't mean that I'd been lunging at them before, but now I didn't appreciate them in the slightest. I believe I'd have greeted Richard Gere strolling naked through my living room with a polite nod and an offer of coffee. I noticed that I wasn't paying much attention to my own appearance, either. I'd never been a clothes-horse, but now I hardly ever looked in the mirror and thought, *Yes. That scarf is smashing with that dress.* I rarely looked into a mirror at all. Or bothered with a scarf. My dreams, which had always been vivid, had also died from the neck down. When I could even remember them, they were devoid of physical pleasure, erotic or otherwise. The more I thought about it, I began to feel that someone had simply pulled the plug on my pleasure centers. They'd gone completely dark.

I finally capitulated and made an appointment with a female osteopath I'd seen a couple of times before. She struck me as a sympathetic and somewhat holistic practitioner who, even if she found my complaint frivolous, would be unlikely to laugh in my face. I drove to her office on a late spring afternoon, wondering even as I sat in the parking lot if I was wasting my money and her time. What, after all, did I expect her to do? Give me a bottle of pills that would resuscitate my sensuality?

That's how I prefaced the conversation: "I'm sure it's only stress, and I feel like a hypochondriac, and I know there's nothing you can..." She cut me off. She began by thanking me for coming in and discussing the issue. She felt that many women suffer (and yes, she did mean suffer) the loss of libido but were reluctant to talk about it or were too quick to accept it as one of those things that must be lived with. She conceded that the root causes are more often than not psychological, but there are also physiological problems that need to be ruled out. She looked downright delighted as she started drawing three tubes of blood, rattling off the panoply of tests she would request: thyroid, cholesterol, estrogen and testosterone levels for starters. (Yes, our ovaries do produce testosterone in small amounts, but when the level drops too low, there goes our sex drive.) In all, she ordered a dozen or so tests. I drove home feeling no optimism that anything would come of it, but at least I didn't feel invalidated or mocked.

I was standing in the kitchen when the doctor phoned back a few days later. "I have good news! Well, sort of good, I guess—the tests showed something interesting. This is the first time I've seen this, and frankly, I'm pretty excited about it. I think we've found what's causing your problem, and no, it's not all in your head. Well, I mean, it *is*, but... Just come in and let's go over the test results."

In the exam room, she presented me with a stack of lab printouts. This much I remember: Each result was presented as a horizontal line graph, ranging from some deficient value to an excessive one. Every single one of my test results was dead-center in the normal range but one: Prolactin. My prolactin level had edged decidedly into the red zone. "What the hell is prolactin?" I asked.

Prolactin is one of several hormones secreted by the pituitary gland, which is located at the base of the brain, squarely between the ears; the hormone's primary purpose is to trigger lactation. From an evolutionary perspective, it's not in an infant's best interest for its mother to conceive again while she's still nursing, so a secondary function of prolactin is— you guessed it—to quash the libido. If the cells that produce the prolactin reproduce at an abnormal rate, creating a non-cancerous tumor known as a prolactinoma, the hormone level rises. (To my astonishment, the male pituitary has prolactin-producing cells, and men with untreated prolactinomas will in fact start to lactate.) Mine wasn't at that level yet, but it was high enough, my doctor ventured, to cause my sexual dysfunction and general malaise. She sent me for an MRI to confirm her suspicions, and there it was—the technician pointed it out with the point of his pen, which was probably the same size as the tumor—a barely visible blip, a few renegade cells that were turning my body into little more than a mode of transport for my head.

If she'd seemed oddly enthusiastic about the case before, my doctor was positively jubilant with this result. She had harbored the suspicion for a long time that a fair number of women suffer physiologically-based sexual dysfunction, but she'd not yet laid her own eyes on a case of it. Best of all, the treatment was straight-forward and effective. A drug called bromocriptine both reduces the prolactin level in the blood, thus eliminating the symptoms, and it also slows the cell division in the pituitary. It's been given for decades to women who don't wish to nurse, and it has a long, solid safety record and no side effects. So in the end, I did in fact leave her clinic with a bottle of pills to resuscitate my sensuality.

This prescription did not have the effect of playing the country-western song backward, bringing my mother and my dogs back to life, salvaging either my job or my relationship. I was still blue, and I was still grieving. You could be forgiven for wondering, since I'd found myself single again, wandering somewhat lost in the post-breakup debris, what use was my recovery?

As the medication kicked in, it became obvious to me that an etiolated libido is not limited to a clitoris that's gone numb. Libido encompasses *joie de vivre*, vibrancy of body and spirit. Riding the elevator to my office one morning, I noticed that a man standing in front of me had beautiful salt-and-pepper hair, and I had the fleeting fantasy of running my fingers through it. It took place in a split-second, and that's where it stayed. A mere whisper of thought. I had no idea who he was; I never spoke to him, but that flash of desire was an epiphany. When had I last felt anything like it? I couldn't remember, but I felt like I'd regained the use of a long-paralyzed limb. I was still in boatloads of hurt, but my recovery restored my capacity for pleasure.

The prolactinoma was not, of course, life-threatening. I could have carried on with it indefinitely as do, for example, people who live with chronic depression—going through the motions, functioning acceptably in most areas of my life (and going through the motions and faking it in bed). Only when the feeling started to return did I realize what I'd lost. I feel blessed to have stumbled upon a doctor who was keen to investigate my complaint, and even more that it was easily treated. I still marvel that a miniscule growth on a pea-sized gland increased the level of a hormone I'd never heard of, and frigidity ensued. Go figure.

If I could share any advice with women whose libido has gone AWOL, it would be this: Don't ignore it; it is a precious thing, and just because you can survive without it doesn't mean you should. If you happen to be celibate, don't say it's irrelevant—your sensual self extends beyond sexuality. Don't blow it off as a function of being too tired, stressed or distracted. Don't blame it on your partner or on your age.

Mind you, it might be any of those things or a combination of them, but if there is an organic problem, no amount of relaxation or counselling is going to cure it. Find a congenial doctor who will check those dozen or so factors that could be culprits. If your regular doctor is dismissive, try another. Just don't let your libido languish in cold storage for the rest of your life.

All that took place about 14 years ago; I'm 53 now and experiencing a completely different adventure with hormones. I expected menopause to kill my libido just as surely as the prolactinoma had, but it's still kicking. I know, because I take its pulse regularly. During the long periods of separation from my current partner, I examine myself for signs of sensual numbness the way a diabetic monitors her blood sugar. Does my pulse pick up when I watch an erotic scene in a film? Does my nose perk up when I notice a man wearing a gorgeous cologne? Can I still bring myself to an orgasm that doesn't feel like a waste of time and effort? Yes? Phew! As time goes on, my fear that I'll long outlive my sensuality begins to fade.

About the Author
Esme Stark

What did you want to be when you were eight years old?

A flying carpet pilot

If you could give advice to your younger self about your orgasm (or your body), what would it be?

Be more patient; treat your body with greater gentleness and care. It's not a machine.

If your orgasm had a voice, what would it say to you about the piece you wrote for this book?

Admit it—you were ready to declare me dead and walk away. Glad you didn't, eh? Here's hoping we've got years together!

Anything else you want to share with the readers?

When I mention Betsy's books, *Autobiography of an Orgasm* and the subsequent anthologies, to friends and acquaintances, they often respond with widened eyes and nervous titters. And every time, my heart sinks a bit more. Why are we so nervous and squeamish about something so fundamental and important? It's becoming acceptable, maybe even trendy, to discuss one's pain openly. Why must we avoid the topic of our pleasure?

FIVE
CONNECTING THE DOTS
by Tracey Allred

"You can't connect the dots looking forward; you can only connect them looking backwards. So you have to trust that the dots will somehow connect in your future. You have to trust in something—your gut, destiny, life, karma, whatever. This approach has never let me down, and it has made all the difference in my life."

—Steve Jobs, co-founder of Apple, Inc.

I never really got this quote until recently. Now I can see how all the twists and turns of life, light and dark, positive and negative, have brought me to this point. I could not have known that the shattering and complete loss of the world I knew would bring me to the point of finding my orgasm and literally bring me back to life with such fervent, vibrant joy and freedom.

Towards the end of 2006 things were going really well, especially on the outside. I had a career; I was making great money and loving the work I was doing. I had amazing, fun friends, and for the first time in my life, my body was in great shape, and my brain could actually recognize it for once. I was also having some little escapades of casual dating and, on occasion, consensual sex. I was looking forward to an incredible new year!

On New Year's Day, all my friends and I went to the Polar Bear Dip at Coney Island, all costumed up for the dive into the ice-cold Atlantic Ocean to wash away the past year in order to start anew. I could never have imagined that the tsunami of my worst fears and then some were about to start rolling in, tossing and tumbling my world into darkness. She rolled in hard, and she was not going to let up anytime soon.

I was set to leave on January 2nd to go to Texas to take my dad to see the doctor, as he had not been feeling well. I came home from being a polar bear and began to pack for my trip when the phone rang. My aunt was on the other end of the line. "It's your father. He was rushed by ambulance to the hospital—he cannot breathe at all. They say it's really bad. We are on our way there now." Through the shock I managed to say, "Please tell him to hold on; I'm on my way and will be there tomorrow." I did not sleep that night.

My father and I had just recently gotten close, opening up to each other over the past few years, especially after my mom's death. After asking him lots of questions, I finally understood where he was coming from and why he was the way he was. He'd been an enigma all my life, even though he was always physically present. We had shared that his mother, my grandmother, was verbally abusive to both of us, and often her ways did not match her religious beliefs that she pounded upon others. It was basically a huge part of the reason we both walked away from the "Charlton Heston" God that we were supposed to fear.

I learned a huge lesson about control on that first night in the hospital with my dad. Late that night, he proceeded to tell me that this was his time. He was going to die. He told me not worry about him at all. He was adamant to the nurse, as well. "Oh, you think so… you think you can control that, can you?" she said.

He told her, "Thank you for all you have done, but it's time I go now." He told me he loved me one last time before putting his BiPAP breathing apparatus back on and dozing off to sleep. The next morning when he awoke, he was furious. Yes, he was mad that he was still alive!

Even funnier was the fact that he was not speaking to any of us, including the nurses or doctor. I suppose he was pissed that "Charlton Heston" had failed him. If you knew my dad, this would definitely make you laugh. It certainly amused his close friends when I called them all the following day to let them know what was happening. I can now see that the lesson of control kept coming up for him as I write this—connecting the dots.

A few days later, on January 7th, I sat with my father for several hours as his breathing got more and more shallow, noticing a peacefulness in him that I'm not sure I had ever seen before. I thought about the gifts he taught me: independence, a business mindset, world travel and great driving skills. I was so grateful for getting to know my dad over the previous couple of years, because those times and talks would eventually be a catalyst for helping me connect the dots in my own life and healing my traumatic past.

As my father took his last breath, a flat line crossed the heart monitor, and I fell onto my dad's chest, crying deeply. Even though I knew deep down it was a false sense of security, the only rock in my life and the only person I felt could protect me was now gone. Thus began my fall down into a deep, dark abyss, after which all the mysterious, hidden parts of myself could untangle, untwist and unravel, so I could try and get back to the person I was actually meant to be.

The tsunami did not stop there. It continued for the rest of 2007 and 2008, bringing more painful scenarios: my favorite, funny great Aunt Bennie died shortly after my dad. I was sued personally and professionally for no reason. I made continual trips to Dallas to handle my dad's affairs and the lawsuit. There was a fire in my apartment building, and my dog and I almost died. My best friend's baby sister died unexpectedly, and then my dog of 16 years died. I let go of my long-term freelance job since I was being pushed out as they laid off others. With all of this, not only was I suffering from burn-out but also the undeniable hidden darkness of depression, blackouts, unworthiness, low self-esteem and self-hatred that came from being abused. It all came rising up, leaving me to feel like the bad sinner girl I was. According to what my grandmother had once told me, I deserved all that was happening.

It brought forth that I had always felt dead inside after the sexual and verbal abuse that started when I was five years old. I was able to cover it up quite well, pretending to wear a happy mask so no one would know what lay beneath. This is when Miguel swooped into my life and caught me completely and utterly by surprise with how easily and effortlessly a relationship could flow. Little did I know that he would be one of my greatest teachers, a lover who opened me up to my body and to the love within myself.

At the end of 2007, Miguel first made his appearance by delivering end-of-year packages to me. I was still working at an office, and since most packages required a signature, he asked me my schedule so he could deliver during those times without me having to make the long trip to the center to pick them up. He handed me his cell number on a piece of paper in case there were any changes. I appreciated that at least one thing could be simple and easy at this point in my life. By the time Christmas rolled around, I was at home, sick with bronchitis and feeling depressed. I somehow managed to make cookies for my super, mailman and all shipping guys. One day I answered the door in my sweats, with oily hair and all the messiness of one who is not well; Miguel had brought me a package, and I handed him a bag of cookies. He was surprised and very appreciative. Later that afternoon, I was coming from the bank, standing and talking with my neighbor, when Miguel saw me and said, "Thank you so much for the cookies! They were the best." There was this wild moment of silence and connection, like everything around us had stopped, and a recognition that to this day I can't quite explain. Oddly, my neighbor picked up on it and said, "What was that?"

"What do you mean?" I answered. "I made him cookies, along with the mailman and our super, and he was thanking me for them."

"No," she said, "the energy so thick between you two that you could cut it with a knife." She picked up on it, too. My response was that he was very kind and really cute, but who knows?

A few weeks later, I caught myself by surprise when I called Miguel after not seeing him around the neighborhood and proceeded to ask him out for a drink. Wait. What? Really?

With my history of sexual, verbal and religious abuse, I wasn't too much into being with men, much less having sex. I found it quite excruciating. I have a confession. Up until this point, I had never had sex sober. I would have to transform myself under the influence of alcohol and/or an alternative personality state, because the agony of guilt and shame associated with the act of sex, along with the hatred of my body, was just too much to bear. I needed to check out of my body in some way.

In my 20s, I became celibate. Sex was not fun for me at all—I equated it with marriage and babies and mixed messages from my childhood. I hated the way guys seemed to treat me afterwards, confusing me even more. I hated sex. I hated me. I no longer had any interest in it, even though I wondered often about the people who didn't want to get married or have babies, then what? I still loved men, but I only wanted them as friends, and I had some great ones. If a guy came on to me, I quickly gave them some story, pushing them far away while shutting my façade of a bubbly personality down immediately. My weight, I hoped, would also help serve as a barrier. As long as they remained in the safe space, we were good.

One way to diffuse dealing with what was going on with me was to pour myself into work. I loved my job working in production for commercials, music videos, TV and film. I loved being on film sets, being with my production family, so I never minded the long hours. As long as I was working, I didn't have to deal with the sadness that always lay just beneath, being hidden by a perpetual "happy" mask or alternative state. I would have worked 24/7 just to avoid feeling or dealing with anything sexual, the flashbacks, the blackouts, or being the bad sinner girl.

Miguel picked me up and we drove to a bar in the neighborhood. We began to talk, asking each other questions as we drank the red wine he ordered. The conversation and being in his presence was flawless. And for once, I don't think it was the red wine, as we both took only little sips here and there. I remember one point where he held up his hand, placed mine up to his to see the size and then it turned it into this beautiful caress of holding hands. As we left the bar, I loved how he immediately took my hand and guided us through the thick crowd, then circled his arm around my waist as he opened the bar door and then again with the car door. Once we arrived at the front of my building, I asked him why he was suddenly so quiet. He gently said, "You make me nervous."

I replied, "Why, because you want to kiss me?" And then I leaned over and kissed him on the lips. Wait. What? Me? That began the hot, parked-car make-out session for another hour. When I walked into my home, I sat on the bed, my body shaking like I have never felt before but in the best way possible. There was a tantalizing tingle, and the words came whispering from my lips, *"What have you done to me?"* I felt something alive within myself.

We saw each other sporadically for make-out sessions over the next five months. There was a certain text where he asked if it would be possible for him to see me in my lingerie! What lingerie, I thought? I looked at what was in my drawers only to see that it was not likely what he was thinking about or wishing for. There they were. Bras with wires popping out, granny panties, period panties and panties stretched out with holes. No sight for any eyes, especially for a man that is turning you on! Off I went to Le Petite Croquet, entering the world of pretty bras that actually fit, with matching thongs and panties. Now I knew what the secret of Victoria was, but without all that padding that I certainly didn't need more of.

The night we went out, I think we both knew we wanted to be with each other. Perhaps I should say, he may have known before, but I was finally ready to have sex with Miguel. My heart was pounding out of my chest, and I felt like I could throw up from the nerves that were racing in my body, as I was sober. I had a small sip of wine and decided I did not need or want it.

I led him to my bedroom and sat him down on the bed, where I proceeded to dance to the music, laughing nervously while sensually undressing with the lights on. Wait. What? I hated having the lights on, because it would show all the flaws of my body that I hated. I somehow used humor and dance to manage the glow of lights to turn us both on. Finally the turn-on outweighed the guilt, shame and body hate.

Miguel took me in his arms, his hands gently moving along my body, slowly kissing my lips and then my neck. It felt so nice, like nothing I remember feeling before. I was lucid and in the moment, with no altered state. As he laid me gently on the bed, eyeing my body, I could see the expression on his face, and it was not one that screamed disgust or slut. And then he said it. "You have a beautiful body, Tracey." And for once, I did not discount him or myself. I took it all in.

I felt a sense of breathless calm as he kissed my upper thighs, and moving them farther apart, he began to worship me with his tongue. I actually felt wide open, alive with connection—something I had never experienced before. An orgasm. And another. Another. I was in the moment, and I could feel them. I was alive. Those tears that slowly formed and fell from the sides of my eyes were of pure gratitude.

As he leisurely made his way up my body, kissing my stomach and then slowing down to pay special attention to my breasts, my body desired so much more. I found myself pulling him up to my lips to kiss him and feel his entire body against mine. As his body entered mine, I felt this energetic force circle through, and the connection was so strong—as I gasped for air, I thought this must be what it feels like to love. Love for my own body that I had hated. Love for the sober present connection with another. Love. It felt miraculous.

I was 42 years old when I finally had sex without being under the influence of alcohol or in an altered state. I could finally make love with the lights on and not hide behind the armor of my body weight that I used to protect me. I had used it to try and stop the abuse at age seven after one of my molesters told me not to get fat like the rest of them.

Miguel made me feel like a desirable, lovable queen; he would be one of my greatest teachers, advocates and lovers. He taught me to treat myself that way as well, which I'm still learning. We continued this gorgeous friendship of loving, learning, healing and connection for seven years on and off. We are still friends who are traveling different paths now, but we feel so much love and gratitude for each other and the gifts we gave and received. I am eternally grateful for this lover who took me deep and loved me right where I was along the way, recognizing that I was not an easy one as I moved through some deep, dark swamps of sadness, anger, rage and mental health issues.

This quote comes to mind when I think of my time with Miguel: "Crawl inside this body, find me where I am most ruined— love me there." – Rune Lazuli

During a break in my relationship with Miguel, I challenged myself immensely when I took an OM class from OneTaste. OM stands for Orgasmic Meditation, a consciousness practice between two people for more connection and pleasure in every aspect of life. A partner strokes a woman's clitoris for a timed 15 minutes with no goal except for both people to connect and be present.

Having a guy stroke my clit for 15 minutes pushed every religious and sexual abuse button I had. I felt anxiety about being in a vulnerable position of partial nudity and having someone lean over my body while touching my pussy. This was a part of my body that had been controlled by others and lost to me as a child, so much so that I could not even bring myself to participate in the end of the all-day workshop. My nemeses— Guilt, Shame, Sinner, Slut and Body Hater—all showed up to wreak havoc.

However, I knew I desired to go deeper within myself to heal and connect those parts that I had numbed and lost during the abuse, challenging myself to try it at least once. I posted on the OM boards, asking for a partner; the responses were so rapid and plentiful that I became anxious. My friend Wendy held my hand through the process. Brian would be the first; the nerves pressed in on my stomach, as I constantly battled the sensation of potential vomiting. When he was late, all of those societal and religious beliefs started swirling my head. Sinner! Whore! Single women don't have sex, and yet I did not run to food, alcohol or an altered state to numb myself beforehand. I tried to stay in the moment, but there was a point where I did check out of my body despite Brian being very gentle and communicative, helping me to stay calm and breathe. Albeit embarrassing, it was another way to connect with a person that would help me open up further to my life source. The practice itself was meditative and did not feel sexual at all. It was another practice that helped me learn to trust, be honest and stand for myself by speaking up for what I wanted.

It was during my fourth OM that I finally felt the essence of my true self. As my partner was stroking, I had checked out of my body. He burst out with laughter, which brought me back to the moment. That's when I felt the joyful laughter come through his fingertip into my clit, up through my belly and open up my throat to release my own burst of laughter. I saw and felt my four year-old self in vibrant, joyous, freedom—playing. It was so clear. I had been searching for this feeling since the abuse started. And there it lay, deep within my clit, hidden and shut down.

When those joyous feelings went away a day later, I felt rage. My body felt like it was on fire, and truthfully, I wanted to hurt someone and have them feel the pain that I had felt when it was all taken away from me.

A few days later, I saw my fourth OM partner at a class, and there was no way to hide what I was feeling, because I had been crying the entire time since it went away again. It was the first time I was that real, raw and open about something so vulnerable and painful to me with another, especially one I barely knew. As the tears streamed down my face while telling him about my OM experience, he leaped up, thanked, hugged and held me. It was a huge turning point in opening myself up even deeper and being in a real, raw, open space, knowing that if I found that place once, there was hope that I could find it again. My four year-old knew she was one with the universe and everything was one, from the tree I played in, to the dogs we had, to the doodle bugs I was mesmerized by, to singing to the blades of grass and more. I saw everything in its brilliance and in such detail then. I was one with it all.

Writing these stories, I was able to connect the dots, and I realized that my father helped conceive me in a state of orgasmic sex with my mother. His death was the beginning of taking me deeper into this journey of my own depths, a journey to heal and a catalyst to help me find my own orgasm that died at age five. Looking backwards, I can now see how every tragedy, person, event and moment helped me find those lost parts of myself that would bring me back to my life source.

About the Author
Tracey Allred

What did you want to be when you were eight years old?

I wanted to be a comedian, entertainer, singer and dancer like those I admired and lovingly watched on TV. Some of my favorite influences were Carol Burnett, Lily Tomlin, Richard Pryor, Johnny Carson, Flip Wilson, Tim Conway, George Carlin, Gilda Radner, Cher, the performers on Laugh-In and the dancers on Soul Train. Comedy, laughter, dancing and singing were a big part of my life, and I think they are truly the things that saved my life as a child. I could get lost with them and pretend a different life. Anytime I could perform Carol Burnett, Lily Tomlin or Gilda Radner skits, whether for family events or on the front porch as my stage and the blades of grass as my audience, I would. I also pretended to be a dancer on Soul Train as I stood in front of the TV set mimicking all of the great dancers. I always knew that I wanted and had to be the boss of many different creations. I was very bossy as a child, and I believe this is where the independence, creating, and being a producer came into my life.

If you could give advice to your younger self about your orgasm (or your body), what would it be?

You, my love, will find your orgasm again. It will be worth every road traveled and better than you could imagine despite some deep, dark challenges. Your life source will continue to grow, finding more pleasure in all aspects of life once you have discovered and continue to nurture you and your orgasm with self-love. Keep exploring and taking risks while listening to your heart's desires. It is all within you, my love.

If your orgasm had a voice, what would it say to you about the piece you wrote for this book?

My orgasm would say you are being very courageous and brave now by opening up and being real, raw and vulnerable about your life, despite being scared what others may think or say. I am proud of you for owning your story, your life, your orgasm and finally giving it a voice. Your own voice.

Anything else?

I went through so many different writings of stories for this book that I was amazed how much was deep within that wanted to come up and speak. I found myself having a challenging time sitting still to write, as the deeper I went, the more I wanted to get up and take a walk or do something different. This is where I knew I needed to stay with the emotion that was coming up and write. There was a lot of emotion surrounding the story around my father's death. I didn't realize how much it was still affecting me; losing him made everything in my life rupture deeply. I believe I had the false sense of security that as long as I had my dad, everything would be ok. And when I was writing about Miguel, I realized how much I truly loved this man and what he meant to me. I think he allowed the game of push-pull I played until he just couldn't do it anymore. I couldn't see it then, but I see it now. The dots have been connected. I have nothing but immense gratitude for all of those dots now.

Six

I Love My Ladyscape

by Lisa Lister

I love my lady landscape.

I love my clit and her 8,000 nerve endings.

I love my 80s style bush which I'm sure would be frowned on by the current wave of 'shave 'em bare' fans.

I love my menstrual cycle (yep, I really do love that each month I get to experience my full cyclic nature as a woman thanks to my period.)

I love the lady magic I make in her: Fire, creativity, orgasms, creativity.

I love the power that is held in her.

Just so you know, this is not how it has always been.

In 2004, after years of pain, trauma and misdiagnosis, I was told I had Polycystic Ovary Syndrome (PCOS) and endometriosis. I finally had a name for what felt like a chainsaw ripping at my insides daily. To paraphrase Ani Di Franco, it felt like my cunt was a wound that wouldn't heal.

If I'm honest, for a moment there I was relieved to finally have a diagnosis. Except when we give a name to things we often give them power, too, and the power it gave the medical professionals at the time was an insta-green light to take out my ovaries and womb in order to cure the pain. In fact, the doctor's actual words were, 'You're not going to be able to have children, so it makes much more sense for us to whip out your whole reproductive organs.'

I can pretty much guarantee he's never won an award for his tact and diplomacy. Or bedside manner. I was in shock. I was 25 at the time, and my boyfriend and I had not had the 'children chat'. When I questioned the doctor, he said, 'Why would you need your womb and ovaries if children are no longer an option? Surely being pain-free is the goal?'

Sure the pain was debilitating; I had to take myself to bed for entire days, and I was forever cancelling meetings, appointments and social engagements. In fact I got myself a reputation as a total flake just because I was too embarrassed to say *I can't come out/to work/to the meeting because I'm bleeding through industrial super-size pads, and my bed looks like a scene from the movie* Carrie.'

I didn't know the incredible power that we hold in our womb at the time, but that day, in that doctor's surgery, SHE awoke in me. A fierce mumma-like rage that meant I simply wasn't going to let them 'whip her out'. I left that doctor's surgery with a handful of leaflets as to what my next steps should be, but instead of reading them, I got geeky and did a lot of research of my own.

I read books, read about other women who have endometriosis—each case was different—and most importantly, I discovered that having PCOS and endometriosis didn't necessarily mean I couldn't have children.

I got mad at modern medicine's quick-fix, 'whip it out' mentality, I also got pretty mad at the boy masquerading as a man who I thought was to be my forever love. For him, the PCOS and endometriosis was just one big, 'bloody inconvenience'. Not only could I not have sex as often as he'd like, when I did it was so painful that I just wanted it over with. It wasn't fun, there were very few orgasms, and there was a sense of ridiculous obligation on my part and increasing disappointment on his.

As you can imagine, this did not a long-term relationship make. He was most definitely not the forever love. He said the relationship broke because I was broken. The relationship actually broke because I broke.

I broke open.

I broke open to the experience of being a woman, and I cried. I cried for me, I cried for my friends, I cried for women who are being abused, raped and who don't have a voice. I cried for mumma earth, who is being abused, raped and doesn't have a voice. I realised that the pain I was feeling in my uterus was the pain of ladykind. I vowed to come into relationship with, and hopefully one day love, my lady landscape.

This declaration to my lady bits took me on an adventure—an adventure where I found myself thanking the goddess for the pain, the PCOS and endometriosis, over and over again, because it bought me home to the truth of who I was. There was the life-affirming bit of the adventure where I went on trips to Paris, ate macaroons, took lovers as if I was Anais freakin' Nin (it turns out Forever Love had been the problem and NOT my lady bits after all), and I went on a six-month dude detox before manifesting a hot Viking who is now my husband and the divine masculine to my divine feminine under the light of a full moon… and then there was the *other* bit. The bit that was spiralling down deep inside me and demanding that I question what it actually means to be a woman.

And I continue to question it. Every single day.

Shit got deep.

I took part in magical rituals, fertility dances and ancient temple arts. I learned how to work in tune with the cycles of mumma nature, the season and my body, had healings from shamans and womb women, danced ecstatically, initiated myself to the Goddess by immersing naked in the White Spring in Glastonbury, drank sacred cacao as a feminine plant teacher, practiced womb and abdominal massage (the ancient art of belly rubbing), ate differently, took all kinds of incredible herbs and tinctures, explored sensual movement and tantric sexual practices to slowly come back into a deep, delicious devotional with my womb. I realised that if I dared to trust her, I could begin to heal my own pain, because while modern medicine is great—it saves lives—modern attitudes surrounding it are not. I discovered that if I reconnected with my body, and more specifically my womb, on a daily basis, if I lavished her with attention and love in the same way an attentive lover would, she would make her own medicine, and that medicine would heal the world.

I call it SHE power: the potent and powerful medicine that's made when a woman really bloody loves her lady landscape.

I have absorbed so much through my sexual centre without even realising it; every person who's touched me intimately has left an imprint—lovers, one-night stands, doctors giving me an examination, people who I didn't want to touch me, uncomfortably tight jeans, the cycle seat in spin class (FYI: I only went once, hated it)—and what I'd received and was continuing to receive didn't feel good. Emotions such as guilt, fear, shame and abuse were stuck in my power portal, my womb space, creating sexual organ armour. This armour protected me from the pain, but it also stopped me from feeling the good stuff. It created all sorts of physical, emotional and energetic symptoms such as repressed anger, depression, blocked sexual and creative energy, frustration, bloating, fear of intimacy and abandonment, low self-worth and self-esteem, feelings of unworthiness and difficulty with orgasm and receiving pleasure in all its forms. The most important lesson I learned on my Love Your Lady Landscape adventure was *to receive*. To fully receive.

I go into schools and colleges, talking to girls about self-esteem, body image and sex education, and EVERY time we talk about sex, self-respect and the act of receiving, girls believe—yep it's actually part of their belief system—that they should be the one giving pleasure, not receiving it, and when I ask them why they give pleasure, they say it's to receive love/validation/proof of existence and worth.

'I need to do well at school to make my parents proud.'

'I'm going to become a doctor because it's what my parents want.'

'I smoke because I want to be cool and for the girls in the year above me to like me.'

'If I give him a blow job, he'll like me.'

'He'll like me even more if I swallow.'

I'd sound the 'this-is-bullshit' horn, but honestly? This just makes me sad.

It makes me sad that I'm STILL hearing this from both women and girls. It makes me sad that with porn being so readily available, teen boys believe every woman's prime goal in life is to satisfy *his* sexual needs by performing reverse cowgirl with body hair removed to within an inch of her life with absolutely no concern as to how to give her pleasure. (And for her to not love herself enough to know what she likes because she's never been taught to receive pleasure, and if she *does* know, she doesn't have the confidence to ask for it.)

It makes me sad that there are women in the world who still haven't experienced an orgasm. It makes me sad that some women will *never* experience an orgasm because their culture dictates that their clitoris is removed.

Loving my lady landscape is a daily practice in:

Reconnecting with my body through movement and touch.

Remembering who I am underneath the armour—a goddess, a priestess, a witch, a healer, a daughter of the great mumma. (This really is a daily practice, because no one wants us to remember THAT kind o' power.)

Reverence for the incredible power portal that lies between my thighs. I worship, cherish and lavish love upon my yoni. I chant to her, I breathe into her, I respect and honour her and all that she represents to me as a woman in the world.

Receiving love and respect from my hot Viking husband who at times represents the patriarchal constructs to which my Shakti, my divine female essence often finds painful to navigate and negotiate, yet he truly worships at the altar of SHE in me, tirelessly and without question, which allows me to receive the lessons, the pleasure, the grit and the blessings that being truly in my SHE power offers up.

About the Author
Lisa Lister

Author of *Code Red: Know Your Flow, Unlock Your Monthly Super Powers and Create a Bloody Amazing Life. Period.*

Web: www.thesassyshe.com
FB: www.facebook.com/pages/Sassyology
Twitter: @lisaclark

What did you want to be when you were eight years old?

I wanted to be a fashion designer. I was obsessed with my Fashion Wheel and made entire catalogues of the same skirt in seven different colours and styles. Think it makes total sense that I now write.

If you could give advice to your younger self about your orgasm (or your body), what would it be?

You deserve to feel good. To feel pleasure. To ask for what you want. Your lady landscape is to be explored and not ignored. Go do it.

If your orgasm had a voice, what would it say to you about the piece you wrote for this book?

She'd then let out a long, delicious pleasure-filled exhalation that she'd finally been felt and heard. Ahhhhhhhh.

SEVEN
PUPPIES AND PUSSIES
by Jane Miller

I wish I knew when he gave me a puppy, there was a leash attached, and it wasn't to the dog.

I met him when I was twenty-five. He was smart, funny and charming—the perfect combination to make me put on my rose-colored glasses for our first date. The glasses allowed me to see only the things I wanted to see.

At first, I resisted his offers to go out, the main reason being that he lived with a woman—his girlfriend. He kept explaining to me that he'd been trying to get her to move out for months. He said they hadn't had sex for years. I felt sorry for him. They lived in separate bedrooms and shared custody of two dogs. One of the dogs was a gift he gave her when they first started dating several years earlier.

After months of ignoring his invitations, including a cheeky message he left on my voice mail telling me he was going to marry me someday, I finally met him for a drink in the early afternoon. We talked for eight hours. I didn't allow him to kiss me at the end of the date, but I left knowing it would happen soon.

We had sex for the first time two months later. It was the week his former girlfriend finally moved out. She took her dog, food from the kitchen and most of his furniture. Nearly all the shelves in the house were bare, but in the medicine cabinet she left her unused birth control pills, and in the closet she left a wedding dress, like a warning for me. My rose-colored glasses were already blurring my vision. He called her crazy, and I believed him.

A few weeks later, he bought me a golden retriever puppy. We named her Murphy. He told me the puppy should live at his house—which was his way to get me to move in with him. I didn't realize it was the first time the leash would go around my neck. A few weeks later, he surprised me with a new car.

We lived together for ten years and had two children. When I found out he was sleeping with my best friend, I decided to leave him. They often walked our dogs together when I was busy with the kids. I just thought she was being a good friend to walk my dogs, not knowing it was really about her pussy. When I found out about their affair, I actually felt sorry for him. He said she had manipulated him. He called her crazy. I believed him.

After my friend, he started dating a woman ten years younger than me, twenty years younger than him. Within the first months of their dating, I spotted her out with a puppy, then a new car, then a diamond engagement ring. He moves quickly. I could see the leash around her neck even if she couldn't feel it.

As their engagement was ending, he got another woman pregnant, and suddenly my kids had a new sibling instead of a new step-mother. At one point my ten year-old asked me, "Who is Dad's girlfriend?"

We were never too sure, but we fell in love with the new baby, and everything looked okay until he bought the new baby's mama a dog—and then I knew it wouldn't last. When they broke up, he called her crazy and, once again, I believed him.

It was several years after our split when our dog Murphy died. Murphy had been riddled with cancer for months, slowly losing control of her vision, her bowels and her legs. The last days of her life, instead of putting her down, I fought to keep her alive. I carried her in and out of the house when she needed to relieve herself. I walked her to the dish of food when she was too confused to find it. I cleaned up after her for two more days until I realized I was doing her no favor by keeping her alive.

I sobbed as I removed Murphy's collar before she was given a lethal dose of medicine. I realized I was finally grieving the end of my marriage, because Murphy was the one to give me unconditional love the whole time I was with my husband. As I loosened her collar, my own neck came free from a leash that had been holding me for fifteen years.

The month after Murphy died, the rose-colored glasses finally came off when I discovered my former husband's affair with our family nanny. The first thing he bought her was a puppy. Then she showed up driving a Range Rover. She has no idea that leash can nearly choke you to death when you are longing to run free—or be loved. Or remember that you aren't crazy, even though that's what he told you for years.

About the Author
Jane Miller

What did you want to be when you were eight years old?

I wanted to be Lucille Ball. She was curious, glamorous but playful, enjoyed having fun with her best friend and had a husband who sang to her and adored her, even at her least lovable moments.

If you could give advice to your younger self about your orgasm and your body, what would it be?

Don't let yourself, your body and your orgasm be bought. Generous gifts, especially at the beginning of dating, can sometimes be substitutions for real love and intimacy.

If your orgasm had a voice, what would it say to you about the piece you wrote for this book?

Writing down your story is sometimes the only way to make sense of your past so you don't make the same mistakes in the future.

EIGHT
HEALING THE HEALER
by Robyn Dalzen

My journey to Ketut, the healer, began in the town of Pemuteran on the northern coast of Bali. I was spending a few days there with a friend after attending a movement retreat in Bali's spiritual capital, Ubud. We arranged a day of snorkeling with a British couple at the same lodging. As we drove to the snorkeling site, we compared notes and travel recommendations for the rest of our journeys.

The couple recommended a location for a traditional Balinese spa and sauna experience. In the evening, I read reviews of the spa online, many of which mentioned "Ketut," his use of a medicinal herbal scrub, and how he had learned the healing arts from his grandmother. It sounded like something worth experiencing.

Upon my return to Ubud, I met up with several other women who had participated in the movement retreat, which was focused on tapping into the wisdom of our bodies, wisdom that is "wise, wild and free." They mentioned visiting a healer named Ketut. Could it possibly be the same man? Ketut is a common name in Bali—like John in the west. But as they described the herbs and sauna, I realized it must be the same man. Surely this was a sign that he was someone I needed to visit.

I wrote down Ketut's contact information and sent him a text message asking if he had time to see me. He offered me a spot at 3 pm that afternoon. I said yes. But there was no mention of a location. I saw on his Facebook page that he had been seeing clients at a café in town, so I sent a message asking if I should meet him there. He replied, "I come get you soon." Not knowing exactly how to interpret his response, I decided I would wait for him at the café.

It was a Saturday afternoon, and the street was quiet as I meandered down the dusty lane looking for the café. When I finally located the place, the shades were drawn, and a sign said in English and French, "Closed on Saturdays." I sat on the steps, took a few deep breaths, felt the warm breeze on my face, and I waited. Several scooters motored by, and with each one I looked and wondered, is that Ketut? Finally, a scooter came to a halt in front of me, and a man with a warm, wide grin looked at me and said, "Hello! I am Ketut!"

We exchanged greetings and introductions, and then he said he would see me at his home, which was a short scooter ride out of town. Was that okay? I checked in with my body, seeking its wisdom and inner knowing that I'd been researching the week before on the retreat. I felt safe, so I said yes. He gave me his helmet, and I climbed on the back of the bike. I asked if it was okay to hold onto him, and his response was, "Yes, please! The tighter the better!" Between bumps and jolts on the ride, he asked me where I was from and what brought me to Bali. I wasn't sure exactly what brought me here, other than a deep knowing in my body that something needed to heal, and this was the place to do it.

As he parked the scooter outside his compound, I removed my helmet and he turned and said in a jovial tone, "Maybe you can kiss me now? Too soon?" His tone was playful and felt harmless, so I returned with laughter and said, "Ketut, you have to earn your kiss!" We entered the compound, which was set up in the traditional Balinese manner with small buildings facing each of the four directions.

We were greeted by two dogs and a pig, which I later learned had been his companions through a recent separation from his wife. They kept him company as he slept alone in his brother's unfinished home. His aging mother sat on the stoop, grinding some kind of powder with a large mortar and pestle. A young girl ran in and out, and several others wandered about as we sat at a table outside his home chatting. As I sat with my thoughts, I felt a slight discomfort not knowing what was next or how this would work. My body, on the other hand, was at ease; it felt calm and ready to allow the experience to unfold.

We sat outside for some time, and Ketut talked as I listened. He told me his story—learning about the power of herbs from his grandmother at an early age and knowing at the age of 12 that he had a gift for healing. But other voices and influences took over, and he decided to follow a more conventional path. It wasn't until years later that he returned to what he knew in his heart was his calling. As he continued to share, he said, "I don't have a piece of paper to demonstrate my skill. I just know what I know." I admired his willingness to leave convention behind and follow what he knew in his heart to be true. I was venturing onto the same path.

Finally he paused and asked, "Why are you here?" I shared with him that I was in a place of transition in my life. I had quit my job two months before, and I was still unsure of what was next. At times I felt joy and celebration and at other times sadness and fear. I had had an amazing career in the environmental sector, facilitating the protection of some of our planet's most threatened species and working with inspiring and passionate young people around the globe. But at some point this career that had fed me began to take my energy, leaving me depleted and burned out. I needed time to regroup, recharge and find my passion again. And then I added a desire to increase my capacity to receive love.

This launched us into another conversation, and Ketut opened up about his marriage, his heartache and his desire to find his beloved— someone who understood him and his calling and was willing to stand by him and support him. After 20 years of a tumultuous marriage and four children, he had recently called it quits with his wife. It was comforting to hear that even Balinese healers have challenges with relationships. He shared that he was ready to find his new partner, and an intuitive friend recently told him that she is on her way to him. With a glint in his eye, he looked at me and smiled. "Maybe it is you?"

It was nearing 4:30 pm when he invited me inside for the healing session. A batik cloth covered the massage table, and Balinese music played softly in the background. As my gaze moved across the room, I saw necklaces with crystals hanging on the wall next to Balinese masks. Glass bottles filled with liquids of varying colors covered the desk, candles and incense were burning and oil was steeping in a broad bowl filled with herbs. This was far from the sterile spa environments I was used to. I changed and lay face down on the table trying to relax into whatever was coming next.

Once I settled myself, Ketut swept across my skin with a bundle of soft twigs, which felt like a clearing of space so he could begin his work. He sprinkled salt across my body and then poured the herb-infused oil on my skin. I felt the oil drizzle onto the table and pool at the base of my back. To top it off, he splashed holy water that cooled my skin. It made me think of a chef preparing a delicacy with his finest ingredients. And then the massage began.

His strokes were deep and deliberate, as if he were clearing away layers of deeply held emotion. He worked on my back and legs and then had me turn over, and he worked his way down to my feet. He firmly pressed into the inside pad of my foot. Ouch! He then moved to my toes, pressing and holding. The pain was excruciating as he moved from one toe to the next. As the muscles throughout my body tightened, the message I heard within myself was to breathe into the pain, feel it and release it. I became more present to the pain and sent my breath through my body down to my feet, but it still hurt like hell.

This was the beginning of his assessment of what needed to heal. After checking the right side of my body and then the left, he lowered my feet back to the table and said my heart, lungs and kidneys were weak. He placed crystals on my forehead, solar plexus and abdomen and began chanting. The healing began. I breathed deeply and tried to relax. He then invited me to join him in chanting OM. Our voices melded together, and the sound reverberated through my body.

At one point Ketut leaned over and whispered in my ear, "You have to forgive. Forgive yourself and forgive others. Leave behind what no longer serves you. Let go of people and things that hold you back." How many times had this come up before? I had spent years in therapy talking about forgiving myself and forgiving others. And I thought I had. But deep down, had I really let it go and released it from the darkest cavities of my body? I started to realize that our bodies have a long memory and are able to store emotion in hard-to-reach places. We have to gently peel away layer after layer until we get to the core. It may take years. It may take lifetimes.

As tears streamed down my cheeks and onto the table, memories started surfacing—the tragic death of my brother 15 years ago; my marriage, which happened shortly after my brother's death; falling into depression and not wanting to go on living; and then the death of my marriage nearly ten years ago. I checked in with myself. After all these years, what else needed to be released at this time?

My thoughts turned to my brother. He had struggled with drug addiction for many years and had attempted suicide several times. His death carried a shock but was not a complete surprise. I often thought his karma was mixed with that of a cat—he'd been given nine lives, which he ran through in only 21 years. My emotions at the time were all over the place, from grief and sadness, to anger and disappointment and even relief. I would no longer have to dread the calls from my mother or father telling me something had happened to Jeff. I didn't know what to do with all these complex feelings, so I locked them away and allowed only sadness to show its face.

Over the years I watched others grieve the loss of loved ones and was touched by the wide array of emotions they felt safe enough to share, as well as the loving ways in which they paid tribute to their loved ones. I had also noticed judgment toward myself for not being better at grieving and not giving Jeff the proper memorial he deserved—as if the grief was not enough.

Rather than losing myself down the rabbit hole, I came back into my body and my breath. With my heart open, I forgave Jeff for leaving me in such a painful and traumatic way. I forgave him for his struggles in life and the impact it had on our family and on me. I forgave my parents for not saving him. I forgave them for not teaching me how to grieve. I forgave myself for my anger toward Jeff. I forgave myself for not knowing how to grieve. I forgave and allowed the pain to wash over me and to heal me.

My thoughts then wandered to my marriage. I had married only two months after my brother died; it was a very rocky start with the dark cloud lingering over us. I tried to push away the dark feelings and celebrate the honeymoon phase of my marriage, but that only exacerbated the problem. Our first year of marriage was a far cry from my childhood fantasies of bliss and joy, and as the hard reality set in, I found myself spiraling deeper and deeper into an abyss.

About three years into my marriage I woke up to my despair and took notice. I found my thoughts drifting one afternoon to a fantasy about death. I imagined peacefully submerging myself in a bathtub and not coming up for air. The thought jolted me awake from my walking slumber. I sought help, and I got better, but I never really addressed the shame I felt for wishing I were dead. As I lay on the massage table in Bali with Ketut chanting over me, I forgave myself for giving in to the darkness. I forgave myself for wanting to die. I forgave myself for giving up on life.

For many years after my marriage ended, I blamed myself for all that went wrong and its ultimate failure. We had both taken turns playing the victim, and I ultimately took the blame and ran with it. It felt easier that way. Again, I took a deep breath and came back to my body as I spoke gently to myself. I forgave myself for the ways in which I acted out from a place of fear, for losing my voice, for giving away my power and for blaming circumstance. I forgave myself for being unfaithful, for losing my center and myself. I forgave my ex for his shortcomings. I forgave him for blaming me. I forgave and allowed the pain to wash over me and to heal me.

The more I forgave, the more open I felt, and a wave of gratitude washed over me. In choices big and small, I had done the best I could. My parents, my brother and my ex had all done the best they could. Life is about making choices and then learning all we can from those choices and using that information to do better the next time. As I came back to the present moment, I felt gratitude to be alive. I was grateful to remember and to feel, so that I could let go and heal.

Ketut began pressing into my feet again. I braced myself. It was still painful, but not quite as bad as the first time around. "Your heart is more open. You have begun the healing," he said. "Let go of the external messages and voices to create space to hear your own voice." He then asked me to repeat my name to myself three times with love and acceptance, letting the sound of my name resonate within my body. I felt a sense of calm and peace. My body was tingling from head to toe. "That is the end of the session. How do you feel?" I told him about the tingling, and he said, "That is a sign that you are coming back into yourself." How much of my life had I spent living outside of myself? If this is how it felt to be in my body, why would I ever leave?

I sat up and tried to reorient myself in the room. I had no concept of time, other than the fading light of day. Ketut sat at the edge of the massage table and asked me about the meaning of my name. He said our name is our link to our ancestral roots, and it is important to remember where we come from. It grounds us. As I considered the meaning of my name, I remembered a time from my childhood when I was asked to write the story of my name.

I had made up a story about how my parents were camping when my mother went into labor. She ended up giving birth to me in the woods, and as I was born a robin flew by. My mother later confirmed that, as a baby born in the Spring, she had been inspired by the robins in her garden. My name is my connection to nature. I have the ability to fly free like the birds; it is a way to remember that I am wise, wild and free. It was the second time on this trip that I was reminded that I have wings to fly, and I should not be afraid to soar.

As I shared these thoughts, Ketut's eyes lit up. "I want to show you something." On the back of the door was hanging a small gift bag printed with a cartoon character of a woman with auburn hair and dragonfly wings. "I put this up just a few weeks ago for her [my beloved]— CHECK!" Ketut drew a check mark in the air, as if I had just filled the first requirement by disclosing that I have wings. He had transitioned back from healer to human.

Within this gift bag was a letter he had written to his beloved. "Will you read it and help me make it better?" he asked humbly. "When the right woman reads it, it will resonate, and she and I will both know that it is meant to be." I told him I was honored to read it. We sat down and went through the letter line by line, and I helped him correct the spelling, telling him as a next step to rewrite the letter with the corrections and place it back in the bag.

As we made our way back into town on the scooter, I felt lighter. My heart was full of gratitude for this unexpected encounter and the exchange of loving and compassionate energy. We rode through the rice paddies in the dark, and Ketut shared that he doesn't usually talk so much, especially about himself, when he meets with clients. His expressiveness had been a little surprising, but I had the sense that he was longing for a listening ear. I asked what inspired him to open up this time, and he said he could feel that I am an honest person with an open heart. I was grateful for the opportunity to listen. I smiled. I was coming back to the remembrance that this is one of my gifts.

We agreed to stop on the way back to my hotel for a bite to eat. We had both worked up an appetite. But first, we made a stop at Tegenungan Waterfall, sitting high above the falls at an overlook. The moon was nearly full and shining its light directly over the falls. There was no sound other than the rushing water. Ketut asked me about my travels, and I shared some of my favorite places, including the Namibian desert, where I have never felt so small and insignificant and humbled by nature's expanse, power and beauty. "CHECK!" Ketut drew another check mark in the air with his finger. His beloved will be a well-travelled woman.

Over dinner I shared with Ketut the unexpected circumstances around my trip to Bali. Thanks to the generosity of a friend, I had been gifted the week-long retreat, and had booked my ticket only three days before traveling. Bali had been calling me for some time, and I never could have guessed that it would unfold in this way. I shared that I hoped to come back again soon, and again I received a third "CHECK" of approval as Ketut motioned through the air. Apparently a friend had told him his beloved would come for a short time, leave and come back. He seemed convinced that I was "the one."

The final stop for the evening was back at my hotel. It had been quite a day and I was exhausted. Before parting ways, Ketut shared: "Yesterday I told myself that I needed to rest today. When I received your text, I thought I needed to see you. I see now that this experience not only helped me rest, but it energized me and gave me new hope. I don't feel so alone." I realized that the healing hadn't only been for me. For whatever reason, our paths crossed at this point in time, and we had both been blessed. I kissed Ketut on the cheek. He had finally earned his kiss. I hoped my presence was a sign that his beloved is on his way to him.

As I continue to process the experience in Bali, Ketut's words echo in my mind and heart: "I teach people how to heal themselves." There were many amazing blessings that came to me on this trip, the greatest of which was connecting with myself. I traveled halfway around the world to a small island in order to come home to myself. Ketut gave me a gift of healing. But what I learned was that he was not actually a healer in the sense of one who made me whole. Rather, he held space for me to heal myself. And in that process, I learned that I, too, have the power to move from human to healer.

About the Author
Robyn Dalzen
www.robyndalzen.com

What did you want to be when you were eight years old?

I have always been a seeker, even from a very young age, and fascinated with the world around me and within me. At the age of eight, I wanted to be an astronaut or a marine biologist. Both professions represented freedom, adventure and a glimpse into the depths and expanse of our existence.

If you could give advice to your younger self about your orgasm (or your body), what would it be?

I would sing her a song about my orgasm…"This little light of mine, I'm gonna let it shine…This little light of mine, I'm gonna let it shine…" I would teach her that the greatest contribution she could make in the world would be to love herself, honor her body and its wisdom, and let her light shine.

If your orgasm had a voice, what would it say to you about the piece you wrote for this book?

Relax, let go and allow yourself to feel all the magic and beauty the Universe has in store for you. You are perfect and whole—always have been, always will be.

Anything else you want to share with the readers?

In sharing this story, I realize there may be judgments about the appropriateness of Ketut's flirtatious behavior and in turn judgments about me for my choice to continue working with him. I considered editing the story and only including the parts that related to my healing experience, but that didn't feel like an honest portrayal of the whole experience, which was about the connection between two human beings and the connection to self.

Bali is traditionally a very conservative and religious culture with a significant amount of time devoted to ceremonies and offerings. The influx of Western tourists has had an impact on this, as many Balinese are now reliant on tourism for their income. In the case of Ketut, I can't speak to the ways in which he has changed as a result of his interaction with Westerners. There could be an entire story on this alone, but this is not the story I am telling.

In this story, my experience was dependent on being able to trust and feel safe. And, perhaps with little credit to Ketut's behavior, I felt safe. I trusted myself, which hasn't always been the case in my life. I was able to open up and allow emotion to move through me. Others may not have been able to get to a safe place with Ketut, and that is okay. I appreciated seeing his different sides—his humanness, and his ability to transcend. By seeing the full range of his humanity, I was able to better appreciate the full spectrum within myself and recognize the profane and sacred in all of us.

NINE
THE BOX
by Kim Shirley

Last year, I ended the lease on my beloved Seattle apartment in order to travel. I went through everything I owned to decide what to keep, gift, or donate. A few weeks in, I went into that far right corner of my closet. The one with the box. The box my best friend knows about; I told her its location and to remove it if anything happened to me so my parents would not have to open this box and see things like lube, condoms (I admit I am uncomfortable typing these words), a book on Kama Sutra, Anne Hooper's *Pocket Sex Guide*, erotica, massage oil, a beautiful peacock feather, temporary tattoos, bedazzling jewels, various vibrators including one that looks like a tube of lipstick given to me by my co-workers when I left to backpack through Asia, a vibrator from a workshop that I never figured out to use...

The thing is, I'm guessing a lot of us have these boxes. And it made me wonder, as a single woman, living in my own apartment, why did I still have this box? Why were these books not out on the bookshelves, mixed in between Marianne Williamson and David Sedaris, heart, humor, orgasm. LIFE? Why were these tattoos unused? Shoved away in a box is not super convenient.

And sadly, why is this box so dusty? Because I shoved this part of my life into the far right corner of my closet, that is why. Because it wasn't mixed into my life. It was relegated to the back, a dark place, as if there were some shame in my body's natural desires to be held, touched, to feel that fire, to experience orgasm, climax, sensation. To feel attraction, connection, communion, sensuality and to do something about it. Sex is so many things; there are so many shades of it, so many elements to explore, just like LIFE. So why was I so comfortable traveling all over the world solo, but not with my sex?

And I realize as I type this—it isn't true. I've done a lot of deep, powerful work to heal my relationships with my body, my womanhood, my femininity, my connections with men, with my sensual and sexual nature. I just haven't talked about it. I kept that part of my journey in the far right corner of my closet. Hidden away. Waiting to be embraced and explored. Waiting to feel safe enough to be brought out into the light to feel loved and adored.

In 2011 I met Caroline Muir in NYC. She is one of the pioneers in the goddess/tantra movement. She is an author, a teacher, a priestess, a guide. She was offering awakening sessions. My body lit up. I didn't know what to expect. I just knew I was a yes. I showed up at the apartment on the Upper East Side where she was working. I was a bit nervous, wondering what was going to happen. Caroline's calm, confident, loving demeanor immediately put me at ease. She explained that I would lie on the massage table, and she would massage my body. The massage would include my breasts. She would then get onto the table and ask permission to enter my vagina with her fingers. Then she'd guide me to various parts of my vagina so I could become familiar with them. I would learn where my g-spot was.

Caroline massaged me. I felt her love and care with each stroke. My body started relaxing, opening up, trusting this woman and feeling sacred and loved. Then she got on the table between my two legs and lovingly asked permission to enter my vagina with her finger. I said yes. The very moment she gently glided her finger into my vagina, I started sobbing. I kept saying "I've never felt safe" over and over again as I sobbed. "I've never felt safe. I've never felt safe. I've never felt safe." Although I had known this at some level, to allow these words, these tears, this energy to move through me was profound. The tears and release lasted about 20 minutes. Then she guided me to my g-spot; she described the inside of my vagina—none of which I remember. What I remember is feeling safe with her. Feeling like this was a rite of passage that I had missed out on. If I were living in a tribal culture, she would have been the wise auntie who, when I was a teenager, would have done this. It would have been a great moment of initiation, of pride, of self-awareness. It would have made me understand the sacredness of my sex, of my turn-on, of my vulva, my yoni, my pussy.

And yet even after this powerful moment of initiation I kept that box in my closet. I didn't know what to do with this power, this wisdom that was not around me in the world. Feeling safe with Caroline was different than feeling safe in the world. It would take several more years of working with sexological bodyworkers, S-Factor dance, Qoya, hiking in nature, moments with men, and books to truly feel safer in the world with my sexuality. It's still unfolding, but that initiation with Caroline was a much needed step in reclaiming the truth of my sexuality, my desires, my orgasm. It was part of what I needed to get my box out of the closet.

So while those items are on their way to Goodwill (you're welcome, Seattle), that part of me is here—embraced, welcomed, profoundly proud, and knowing that it is something I need. Let's be honest, it's something the world needs. We need a world where women are reclaiming healthy turn-on, sacred sex, primal truth. All of this lights up the world; all of this creates more communion with ourselves, our earth and each other.

This year at Burning Man I volunteered to "work" at a kissing booth. I had a megaphone with which to play with passers-by and call them in, and a booth with a deli-esque menu of kisses to choose from: passionate, playful, loving, angry, creepy, tantric, grandmotherly, with sides of nuzzle, nibble, fondle and spank. Men and women came up asking for a passionate kiss with a side of nuzzle, or a loving kiss with a nibble. I would choose where to kiss, which honored my turn-on. With each person that came up, some leaning in and raring to go, I asked them to put their arms out at a 90-degree angle, and then I caressed them. I got them grounded, centered. I gazed into their eyes and breathed with them, creating this connection between us. I got a sense of their energy, of what they needed, of what I felt comfortable with, of what turned me on with each person. I caressed beards, ears and collarbones. I kissed chests, foreheads and lips. I whispered words of love. I put my hands on hearts, necks and chests. I used my turn-on and desires to commune with each person. One wife came up for her own passionate nuzzle after seeing her husband receive it. "That was so hot." And it was. It was hot, and I was creating it. I was owning my turn-on and sharing it with the world, helping others get in their turn-on, too. Then all of us took that out into the world, feeling more connected, more grounded and more joyful.

I desire to take this kissing booth energy out into the world. I imagine it on Wall Street. How would it benefit everyone to get back into their bodies and turn-ons while making those trades that have such impact on the world? Investment bankers should get back in their bodies before financing companies that change the world. What if by sharing my turn-on I was able to help others get back into their hearts and bodies and make choices from this place? Living in turn-on changes the game; it goes against the rules of keeping that part of our lives separate from life out in the world.

It's the very thing I've been most afraid of: the power of it, the depth of it, the resistance to it, the fear of it. 5000 years of killing and shaming women for their turn-on—this power and the unconscious shaming so many of us grew up with certainly had something to do with my fear. Now I know my wisdom, my power and my beauty are in claiming and living my turn-on. No more boxes. No more hiding. I proudly, delightfully, gratefully take this SACRED NATURAL part of me out in the world with me, to help guide me, to light me up, to help light up the world.

About the Author
Kim Shirley
www.kimshirley.coom
www.reclaimyourwild.com

What did you want to be when you were eight years old?

I wanted to a fairy godmother and spread love all over the world. And an actress.

If you could give advice to your younger self about your orgasm (or your body), what would it be?

I would tell my younger self that my orgasm is so precious and so powerful. To pay attention to what it was saying to me. To be curious and to learn all I can about my body and my turn-on. To know that it is my birthright to receive pleasure, to get my needs met and to spend time learning what those needs are. That my orgasm is awesome.

If your orgasm had a voice, what would it say to you about the piece you wrote for this book?

Thank you for writing about this and setting me free. Thank you for being so brave to post this on Facebook for all to see. Thank you sharing more and more of our truth. Thank you for honoring me. For valuing me. For reclaiming me. Now let's use all the energy that was in that box out in the world!

TEN

BEYOND THE CLASSROOM AND INTO THE CURRICULUM OF ORGASM

by Dr. E. Powell

Heading south in my blue Honda civic towards the middle of nowhere Virginia in May 2010 to begin my doctorate, I blasted the radio as loud as it would go. With windows rolled down and the ombré gray and blue of the Blue Ridge Mountains fading in the distance to my right, the last thing I was focused on was my orgasm. In fact, had someone asked me at that time whether I'd even had an orgasm, I would have rolled my eyes and cocked my head to the side. "Why all this talk about what goes on under my skirt and pants? Don't you know I'm all brains?"

For the better part of my existence, taking a dive into the sensual unknown was at the very bottom of my to-do list. School had always been my first priority; I thought that studying hard and getting good grades would unlock the key to my independence, living the good life and experiencing the American dream.

School was also how I escaped the harsh realities of my adolescence. My father, a drug addict and alcoholic, abandoned our family when I was

77

ten. My mom, who struggled with schizophrenia, was bitter and resentful. She often projected her devastation onto me, because I was the spitting image of my father and a sorrowful reminder of the man she loved but could not have.

I escaped the chaos by taking refuge in books and school. School was a safe haven and a structured environment—the one place I could succeed, enjoy a little bit of peace, laugh with friends and manage to make both parents proud. My teachers adored me; my report cards always contained notes praising my kindness, good citizenship and thoughtfulness.

However, the older I grew, I could no longer disconnect from my body by channeling all my energy and effort into my brain. The arguments with my mother started when I was around 11, and they grew stronger and more frequent. When I became a teenager, I longed to hang out with friends; I begged to go to sleepovers and birthday parties and to be allowed to walk the mall unsupervised. Even though boys were off limits, I began to take interest in them and they in me. This drove Mom even more insane. She criticized everything from the way I talked to the way I walked, down to the colors I painted my nails. In her mind, even a kiss from a boy could propel me into teenage motherhood. We fought like two alley cats. After one particularly bad fist fight, I left with nothing more than my glasses and the clothes I had on that day. At 16, I left in search of something—anything—that was better than the home I had been born into.

Disconnected from every part of my body except my brain, I spent the next few years accumulating degrees, accolades and work experiences as if they were Girl Scout badges. When it came time for college, I earned a baccalaureate in anthropology. Ever the overachiever, I minored in biology and took up a concentration in Latin American and Iberian studies. Then, I went to work as a teacher while simultaneously pursing a master's degree, obtaining three teaching certificates and running a quilting class for homeless women. After five years, I got tired of the daily grind of classroom teaching and took a huge leap of faith into the unknown around the time that the markets crashed in 2008. That year, I worked ten jobs in one year to make ends meet until I got a big break as a full-time project coordinator in DC. My restless spirit got the best of me, and I headed back to school, deciding that earning a doctorate degree was the only way I could achieve the American dream.

A few months into my doctoral program, I began to receive the first in a series of wake-up calls that I was more than just a brain. The caller, I would later learn, was my orgasm. This wasn't the traditional orgasm that I'd learned about in school, typically defined as a peak or climax during sex. This orgasm could express itself inside the bedroom as a sexual experience, but it was also a deeper, wider, more comprehensive life force—an energy that I experienced beyond the bedroom and, more importantly, in my body. This orgasm was fed up with living life as one big series of accomplishments. It had no more patience with the emotions and sensations that I'd shut down due to the trauma and chaos of my childhood.

The first call reached me where I'd spent the most time hiding—in my head. It came in the form of a breakdown. Grad school is a place where you either go crazy or learn the coping skills that you need to work with your particular type of crazy. When I began my coursework, I hit a huge wall and fell apart. Something inside me was sick of being the good girl, the brainiac, the overachiever. All my life I'd harbored a secret desire to do creative work, like making movies, websites and games. I'd found a discipline that allowed me to tinker with those passions, but the degree still required me to research, analyze, evaluate and publish. It wasn't that I couldn't do the work—I just didn't *want* to do it anymore. For the first time ever, my life experiences became more important than my accomplishments or how much I worked.

Depressed and devastated, I toyed with the idea of quitting the program, but broke and simply out of energy to build myself back up, I resigned myself to stay. In my spare time, I joined a theatrical arm-wrestling group that specialized in challenging social norms. In my debut act, I paraded the stage decked out in gold as FoXXXy Cleopatra, a modern-day take on a 70s legend. Waving to the cheering crowd, blowing kisses, flirting with participants, and connecting to a creative community began to lift my spirit. There was no accomplishment or trophy to take home except the sheer delight of being fully rooted in the experience. This, in hindsight, was an initiation to the realm of my orgasm.

Little did I know that initiation would not suffice. Orgasm would come knocking at the door with yet another wake-up call. By my second year of graduate school, I had stabilized to a degree; I no longer lay in a heap, sobbing on the floor for hours at a time as I had done during the first year. I found a few academic projects that interested me, and I was learning to integrate my social and academic lives, but something was still missing.

This time the call came through the unlikely form of a small, pink book by Regena Thomashauer—*Mama Gena's School of Womanly Arts: Using the Power of Pleasure to Have Your Way with the World*. It had sat on my floor for months, on loan from a friend. To this day, I still don't know what motivated me to pick up the book and actually start to read it. Perhaps sheer boredom during a winter recess, an act of rebellion against the Ivory Tower, or the mere fact that my friend had asked for her book back, which led me to pick it up and begin reading.

Regardless of the reason, that book became my personal pink bible and changed the way I experienced life. Regena's work was appealing on so many levels. It talked about everything that had been off-limits, taboo, and/or suppressed since my childhood—flirting, sensual pleasure, beauty and men. Her writing uncorked the very things that had been lost or stuffed at the bottom of my own Pandora's box. Most importantly, her writing challenged me to venture deeper into my orgasm by allowing myself to desire and to take pleasure in my existence.

Excited that I could want more for myself than diplomas and that life could actually be enjoyable, I dared to venture further, but I didn't know where or how to begin.

Fortunately, when you're too much in your head or too busy to connect the dots for yourself, life will often connect them for you. Indeed, that small, pink book spurred a series of changes that continue to have an impact nearly three years later. Reading and doing the activities helped me experience the first pangs of joy and contentment that I had ever felt in my life. I landed my first boyfriend in four years. School became one of the many ways I expressed myself, not my sole outlet.

One day I flipped over my little pink book and discovered that Regena has a website. I spent the morning exploring every blog post, testimonial and course offering on it. By noon, I worked up the nerve to call her business office, and after discussing the options, I enrolled in the Virtual Pleasure Bootcamp. For the next eight weeks, I immersed myself in teachings that would awaken me to my sensuality and experience as a woman.

That class led me to a retreat in Miami with Mama Gena and other women who had taken her programs. There, I saw and experienced a side of myself that was outside of the books, the brains and academics. Throughout the retreat I connected with amazing women from all over the world. I also stayed on a yacht, which was unheard of given my graduate student salary, and I also scored mega deals at every store I shopped at. To top it off, I won a discounted slot in her Mastery program. That one course led me to the seat of my orgasm. And by entering my orgasm, I mean more than just acknowledging its presence or solely experiencing it through sex. I mean fully inhabiting it, exploring its depths and committing to live in this divine state that is uniquely mine—mine to express and experience in this world at this very moment.

Realizing that I was capable of going even deeper into my orgasm occurred for the first time in the Mastery classroom. About three quarters through the course, I hit another turning point and wake-up call for my orgasm. In this activity, participants tune into how it feels to receive pleasure from another. We then learn to take in even more pleasure by bestowing pleasure on someone else. With dimmed lights and classical music playing softly in the background, I experienced the soft touch of a feather stroking my skin. I slowed down enough to savor the taste of a strawberry touching my lips and whipped cream sliding down my throat. Through this activity, I learned to savor every bittersweet note of a Hershey's kiss.

At the end of the activity, Regena asked for questions and impressions. I had been a quiet participant for most of the course. I had done the homework, used the tools and strategies that she taught and would occasionally brag about some of my accomplishments. However, this time my hand shot up high. I was all the way in the back of the room, but Regena saw it go up from the stage where she stood and stared straight at me. A microphone was soon placed in my hands. Tears streaming down my face, I could barely speak. "Mama Gena, I thought I had been one of those broke bitches who couldn't feel anything." I continued to explain that I had experienced so much in life yet I was numb to the pleasurable parts of my existence and could only feel sensations such as pain, misery, sadness, and disappointment. I had spent years using my brain to block out the pain of my past. "My brain became my path to freedom while I had become a prisoner in my own body. Liberating my orgasm through this activity helped me discovered the freedom in my body (and life) that was a direct result of feeling pleasurable sensations. Feeling that first drop of pleasure was like receiving the gift of me to me."

Surrounded by 200+ women in a small auditorium in NYC, I had actually experienced the tip of my orgasm. For the first time, I felt it in my body and not in my head as I'd experienced everything else. Until that point, I'd gone through the course like I did most parts of my life—never feeling the pure, pleasurable sensation of my experiences and accomplishments. The spark of life that I'd been chasing after in books, degrees, international adventures, jobs and men was right there inside me, waiting to be experienced.

That feeling was a warm, delicious drop of pure pleasure that spiraled throughout my pelvis and expanded like sun rays through the rest of my body. For once, I felt at home in my body and not just my brain. I finally felt fully connected to that life force that had been shut down due to the childhood abuse, neglect, abandonment, and the genuine fear of living life well. I entered that space inside myself that had been forbidden for lifetimes or at the very least since the time of Adam and Eve.

The first taste propelled me to many more explorations of my orgasm. After Regena, I discovered Nicole Daedone's Orgasmic Meditation (OM) practice, which opened me up to experiencing and holding as much sensation of my orgasm in my body as possible. For 15 to 30 minutes a week, I lay on the floor with my legs butterflied wide open as a man stroked my clitoris. During this time, my attention was directed towards the sensation of his finger on the point of contact and how I experienced that sensation in my body. I used my words to make requests to alter the sensation in ways that were pleasurable to me. At the end of the session, my partner and I shared a few words about our experience.

Each OM was unique and unpredictable. Sometimes I felt absolutely nothing and struggled to stay focused and connected with my partner. Other times I saw colors and experienced feelings of depth and lightness, all in a span of 15 minutes. One time, the sensation was so high that my jaw went numb, and I felt such strong jolts of electrical current passing through my body that I worried I was having a stroke. Through this practice, I learned how to recognize pleasurable sensations as I experience them in my body and how to use my voice to make requests for more pleasure.

Ever the eager learner, I continued with my studies and went on to take life-altering classes with the highest paid dominatrix in NYC. She taught the energetic principles behind every exchange. Her work revealed how subtle shifts in voice, behaviors and actions could land me in a submissive or dominant role. Neither role was inherently bad or good, but either could be leveraged to accomplish a particular goal or outcome, depending on my desire. Having previously been on an accelerated track to get as many degrees as I could, get a great job, become a career woman before turning 35, never have to rely on my parents again, and live the American dream, I was now on a fast track to learning all that I could about my orgasm.

As usual I was being the good student, but I quickly discovered that there's only so much that can be taught about orgasm. Orgasm is an experience of direct participation; you don't learn by observing from the sidelines or doing armchair research. When it's had enough of classroom instruction, orgasm will push you in the direction of change, expansion and direct participation. Quite simply, shit gets real—really real and really quickly.

In my case, when my orgasm beckons me to change, to create a new role for myself or to expand to the next level, there's usually some catastrophic wake-up call—I run out of funds, have a major health crisis or experience some profound shift in my thinking that is preceded by deep internal questioning. This time around, I experienced a combination of all of these. In a matter of months, I broke up with a guy that I had fallen for, came down with mono, realized that I was $5,000 in debt, hadn't saved enough for my taxes, still didn't know what to do with the doctorate I had recently earned, and began to question why the bulk of my budget was going to personal development courses. I had hit a dead end where I could no longer pay to study my orgasm; I had to commit to living in and from it.

It was at this breaking point that I realized that orgasms must be experienced and lived. Entering my orgasm simply meant that I acknowledged and allowed myself to experience and feel every last drop of my existence. These courses had provided a framework to understand the mechanics of my orgasm and to discuss the magic of what was going on inside and around me, but I still needed to live, love and experiment with my orgasm. I had learned how to experience my sexuality through these courses, and they opened me to the experience of life by making me conscious of sensation in my body. However, there comes a point in every perpetual student's life where they must hand over the reins to their orgasm and commit to using the classroom of their own life to connect with their own truth and inner mysteries so that they can step into the full power of their orgasm and essentially learn to dance, flow and journey with the endless cycle of their creation.

That journey began for me with 17 days to go until my 33rd birthday. Entering the sacred grove of my orgasm on my own and outside the context of a classroom transformed my life. The night that I entered, I howled with the pain and despair of a breakup but simultaneously found pleasure in reclaiming my right as a human being to feel hurt and love so deeply while sobbing in my sunroom. I entered it again during the recent Venus Retrograde when I rolled on the floor covered in money and danced seductively in my apartment surrounded by candles to call in abundance like never before. Little had I known it, but I entered it the moment I left home at 16, along with the moment that I buried myself in books and school. All of this was part of the experience of my sacred existence—my orgasm.

I enter anytime I give myself permission to feel whatever I'm feeling at any given moment and then consciously choose to make adjustments that allow me to feel the pleasure even more, or to have another sensation of my choosing. I enter the sacred landing of my orgasm anytime I realize that this is my life to create, and my truth is mine to experience and express in the world. I enter it when I ask the Divine to work with and through my creations to take me and the world higher.

Since I left the classroom behind and began an independent study of my orgasm, I've discovered that she is slow, steady, gentle and deep. No longer am I waiting for a teacher to instruct me in what to do, to provide a framework or to show me how to respond. No longer am I constrained by textbook definitions or societal norms around my experience.

I now listen to, flow with and interpret the experience of my existence. That is my orgasm. I've learned to sense and feel her total contradictions. She enjoys the calm stillness of a quiet night with only the sounds of chirping crickets and the occasional whoosh of a car passing down her street. She equally enjoys the cacophony and bustle of a street fair. She enjoys the crystal-clear depth of tonight's super moon. She revels in light but is comforted by the darkness of a candlelit room when she comes home from a long day of work. She relishes every detail, from the spark of her lighter when the flame strikes the wick of her favorite candle to the jingle of her bracelets—each of which tells a story from a chapter of her life. She loves deep, soul-quenching belly laughter brought on by random shenanigans or crude, witty humor. She is a seer who studies the tarot and dances in ecstatic circles like a whirling dervish. She is turned on by creativity and romance. She draws strengths from the trees and is energized by the ocean.

She is so much more than words can capture on a page. She is the night. She is the moon. She is dawn. She is the morning sun. She is the lightning and thunder that signal the beginning of a storm. She is a witch. She is a mystic. She is a gypsy. She is the force beyond force. She is breath. She is life itself. She is that expansive, warm, tingly feeling in my pelvis that purrs "Damn, it feels great to be alive, and it's good to be me on this day, at this hour, at this minute, and at precisely this second."

Breathe. Pause.

Release.

Give gratitude.

Take in as much as you can.

Now, expand and amplify that sensation.

Orgasm.

She is I. I am she.

Brain and body operating as one.

That's how it's always been.

That's how it will always be.

About the Author
Dr. E. Powell

What did you want to be when you were eight years old?

I wanted to be everything from a teacher to police officer to an artist.

If you could give advice to your younger self about your orgasm (or your body), what would it be?

Your body knows. It is the strongest oracle you'll ever consult. Pay attention to how people, places and things make you feel. Then, follow the things that feel good and expansive in your body. Take action on those things and don't spend your time on energy that drains you.

If your orgasm had a voice, what would it say to you about the piece you wrote for this book?

I've been trying to get a hold of you for years and I am so glad you've finally answered my call. The sky is the limit and there's no turning back now. Now that you've entered, let's go deeper and higher than ever before.

ELEVEN
REMEMBERING WHO I AM
by M.R. Gonzalez

Are you kidding me?

Outrage and disbelief—that was my first reaction to what my husband was saying. Then there was a brief moment of doubt, immediately replaced by indignation. How dare he try to pin it all on me?

It felt like a nice and safe place, with the plushest and softest couch surrounded by expensive artwork and fancy diplomas, decorated in soft beiges and creams. The decorative pillows on the couch were fluffed to perfection. Everything about the place felt very inviting until my husband opened his mouth. I thought that by sitting there in therapy we were headed in the right direction. I thought we would be able to work through our issues, strengthen our fifteen years together and turn them into forever after. My husband sat at the other end of the couch we were sharing, telling his version of the problem as the therapist listened. He was imploring, doing his nice-guy routine and acting like the victim, trying to elicit sympathy from the therapist. His mannerisms were that of a three year-old boy explaining why he ate all the candy and blaming everyone else, including his mother, for setting the candy out in the first place. So what was his complaint? "The sex was not good," and that was the reason he was unhappy with our relationship.

Really? That's the best he could come up with? I had a whole list of issues that I was willing to work through if he were truly committed and willing to work on our marriage. How could he just sit there and use sex as an excuse? As he kept talking, all I wanted to do was punch him in the face. How could he sit there and lie, especially since we'd been having round-the-clock, rock star sex? I'd made several shopping excursions down to St. Mark's Place in the Village; I'd bought a few items, including a very sexy and revealing nurse's costume, with which we thoroughly enjoyed role-playing. There were also the props and toys from Toys in Babeland, and we had just been to the ultra-luxurious Mandarin Oriental Hotel in Miami and had experienced our first extended massive orgasm, which had left him speechless. So his comment was a bit of a surprise.

Even though I knew this was an excuse to blame me and to justify his philandering, there was still a tiny part of me that wondered if there was any truth to it. Shortly after that session, the marriage ended. The divorce happened. Looking back, I realized that I was trying to hold onto our marriage, even though I had outgrown it. We no longer had the same views, and maybe we never had. Maybe I was too busy trying to be the perfect wife, mother and daughter that I ignored our differences. Maybe I was trying to do all the work of getting us to a better, more fulfilled life, but not all the participants in the marriage were interested or willing. In the end, it wasn't that the sex wasn't great but that there was no connection or intimacy. How could there be, when he was deflecting all my suspicions and questions and lying to me? Without honesty, intimacy and connection cannot exist. Eventually, I checked out from a sense of disappointment and betrayal, because I had not been respected and honored as our vows had promised. And because I had not respected and honored myself and my voice.

My voice.

My voice had always been strong and determined, questioning and fighting for what was fair. In high school and college we are encouraged to have different views and expressions; at least that's how it was for me. I was surrounded by different cultures, views, opinions and ideas. I went to high school and university in Manhattan, and I loved all the expression of

90

self and acceptance of being different that I experienced there. It was ok to be this way during my schooldays, but once I was out in the "real world," I'd have to conform to society's expectation of a good woman and wife. This was the subtle and sometimes not-so-subtle message I received and that I still see perpetuated in some cultures today. So, I let my voice be eroded, little by little and year by year, until I placed myself on a path of self-reclamation. Then everything changed. I remembered that I had a voice, and I had a right to express it loud and clear. I had a right to be an equal partner in our marriage; I did not have a lesser role just because I was not the breadwinner in our household. I had the right to my opinions and desires. I had the right to voice my desires in the bedroom, as well, and there, they were welcomed without question. It was when I voiced my opinions on how to run my life that I was a potential danger.

There were many instances, although subtle, that reminded me I was not seen as an equal in our marriage. I still remember two of them vividly.

According to my ex, his money was my money. I had stopped working outside of the home to raise our daughter. In theory, I had access to the money, but I had to ask permission if I wanted to purchase large-ticket items. At first I was checking in with him because it was our family finances, and I thought nothing of it. But when he kept buying golf clubs whenever he pleased and went on golf excursions or boys' trips at a moment's notice without consulting me, it felt unfair. If I wanted to buy a purse, it had to go through him. He would resist at first and then he would give me the yes. It felt like he was rewarding me for being a good girl. When he decided I could buy whatever I wanted with no resistance from him, something was up. I just didn't know it at the time. Only later, I realized that he treated me to extravagant shopping sprees when he felt guilty for doing something bad, usually stepping out on me. At the time, I felt I had no say. When I wanted to use the money for something, he reminded that he busted his balls working and that we should be saving. When he spent his money, he seemed to forget about saving. His view was that, as a homemaker, I really didn't do much. He felt he did more because he was the one that brought home the money; therefore I had a limited say in the finances.

I also realized that I was being discounted on the day my ex agreed to loan the car to a friend while he was away without even consulting me beforehand. He called to let me know that his friend would be passing by for the car keys. Excuse me?! He didn't even bother to ask me if I was going to use the car. He balked when I told him no. I told him to call his friend back and say no; if he came around, I would not give him the keys. He was furious—he preferred to look good to his friend than accept that he had disrespected me. Even if I sat home all weekend and went nowhere, I was not going to budge. No more.

The blinders came off, and when I saw the lack of respect I'd been afforded for years, my marriage unraveled. It gave me the strength to leave and make a new life.

When I met the Italian, as I like to call him, I had recovered and moved on. I had made a vow to myself to stay vocal, to always state what I desired and walk away whenever my voice was being diminished or ignored. The Italian was immediately drawn to my innate femininity and sensuality and my lack of inhibition when we were intimate. I was struck by his deep voice and evident masculinity. He was actually half-Italian and half-Spaniard. Six feet tall, muscles everywhere, athletic and a good dancer, with an olive complexion and the most gorgeous piercing green eyes. He was born and raised in Europe; he spoke four languages and was an avid kite surfer. He had abundant stamina and raw sensuality. I was fit, strong and extremely confident. I was a little bit of an adrenaline junkie. I had taken up surfing and helicopter flying and had signed up for race-track time. I had also become a regular in my local salsa scene; I was dancing at least five nights a week, either taking classes or at dance socials. I met the Italian at one of the swanky and hip South Beach hotels. After the preliminaries of meeting and courting, we fell into a rhythm of scorching hot, unconventional trysts.

I remember one particular day when he called to ask if I had "those boots." I knew the kind he was referring to, but I played along. He asked,

"Do you have the boots, you know, the ones that are long? What are they called?"

I answered, "You mean thigh- or knee-high boots?"

"Yes!"

I told him I did have black knee-high boots and asked him if he wanted me to wear them later. "Yes!" he replied. Mind you, it was the middle of summer in Miami. Instead of complaining or thinking it weird, I actually felt exhilarated, and so I took it further. I cheekily answered, "Sí, mi capitan; anything else you would like me to wear?" That got a laugh out of him. He didn't care what else I wore as long as I was wearing the boots. He told me he was going to have champagne and strawberries for me because he knew they were my favorite. A night of delights was ahead and I couldn't wait!

As I was driving home to prepare, I was visualizing different outfits and props to take to his place later. I thought of showing up in a long coat, knee-high boots and nothing else, but it was too hot, and how was I going to pull off walking all the way to my car in that outfit without melting from the heat and humidity? But as I let my imagination run wild, a clear picture started to form. I got home, packed the long, leather tassel whip, the small whip, a black silk agent provocateur blindfold, a long fuchsia feather boa and other sensual paraphernalia. Nothing like planning a tryst to get me all warm and fuzzy.

It was so much fun walking in knee-high boots in the middle of summer while being stared at. I had a secret, and maybe people knew, or maybe they just thought I was weird. All the more fun. When I got to his place, the first thing he did was look at my feet. Boots were in place, check! He smiled mischievously until he saw the complete outfit hiding underneath my form-fitting dress. I was dressed head-to-toe in what looked like dominatrix gear. Black knee-high boots, black thigh-highs with lace trim securely attached to the black lace garter belt that barely covered the black lace thong. And the pièce de résistance? The black leather whip in my right hand, snapping in the air. I thought his eyeballs were going to pop out of their sockets. I just winked back at him as he looked me over once, twice and a third time. Then he became positively primal.

I barely made it inside the door. He unbuttoned his jeans, and to my surprise he was not wearing any underwear. There was something so raw and sexy about that—it turned me on even more than I already was. As the jeans slid down his strong, muscled thighs, he pulled me up, and I wrapped my legs around his waist as I mounted him. He was ravaging me right there in the middle of the living room with no walls to hold us up. He was using his sheer strength, will and passion to make passionate love to me with no support other than our bodies. As I was moving up and down to a delicious but frantic rhythm, with each rise and fall moving us closer to exquisite release, I slowed us down. I wanted to savor the moment and move to the bedroom where we could take our time. And savor every moment we did. There was not one inch of our bodies that wasn't caressed, nibbled, licked, whipped or sucked to delirium. I felt uninhibited, wild and carefree, completely in my body, taking in every moment, not rushing to completion or with an end-goal in mind. It was wild, free, passionate and tender. All these things I knew were inside of me, but I had almost let my ex-husband's words plant the seed of doubt in my mind. This particular sensual encounter and this passionate love affair reminded me of what was inside me all along.

Many orgasms later, we were satiated. Leaving the bed, on his way to the kitchen, he stepped on a small black whip with a pink feather tip. He looked at the floor, which was littered with the black silk blindfold, scattered pink feathers and other items, and he grinned, shaking his head in disbelief. Pointing towards the floor, he said "No one has ever used that on me before." I just smiled and did a silent fist pump in my mind. I had successfully introduced sensual toys to a man who had never explored them until he met me, and he was in his early 40s.

I followed him to the kitchen to drink the champagne and eat the strawberries he had gotten for me. He hand-fed me strawberries by the open fridge while I stood there in black thigh-highs, garter belt and black knee-high boots as if I were wearing regular clothes, feeling completely comfortable. He asked me, "Are you always like this?" He was actually asking if I'm always comfortable with the lights on, wearing lingerie and not trying to hide my body, open to exploring and very clear about what I like, want and don't want.

"Yes," I said.

He furrowed his brow and shook his head and said, "I don't understand why you got divorced." I just nodded with a sly, sexy smile, agreeing with what he was thinking. With that one sentence, he was asking how come a beautiful, smart, sexy, funny and uninhibited woman who can articulate her desires and fulfill his, is divorced? He was implying that I was the whole package, and if he were married to me, he would not have let me go. He would have done everything in his power to make me a happy woman. And in that moment, I knew and felt it in my core that I have always been one hot, passionate woman, and it was never about my sexual prowess.

Since the Italian had a strong character, he was unwavering and clear on what he wanted; he could be intimidating. Even in the bedroom he was used to dictating what he wanted, but not with me. From the start, I established that I was also going to be participating, and not only with my body but with my mind, my desires and my voice. I let myself be outrageous in my demands. We went head to head in the bedroom as well as outside of it, but always with humor. I always felt my power. I felt strong, secure, determined in my voice and femininity. I felt like a fully embodied woman. This reemerging power gave me the strength to move on when our time together was complete without staying a moment longer, as I had done with my previous relationships.

It reminded me that I have always been of strong character. When I lost myself for a while, I had allowed the outside voices, the world's opinions and even the voices of my loved ones who meant well, to dictate what my life should look like, even inside the bedroom. Sometimes when I feel that my thoughts are slipping in the direction of conforming to someone else's standards, I ask myself, "Do they pay your bills or take care of you when you are sick? NO! So why do you care what they say? Why are you trying to please them?" This brings me back from the edge and to the woman I am—a woman who derives her strength and her femininity from her unwavering voice.

About the Author
M.R. Gonzalez

What did you want to be when you were eight years old?

Wonder Woman

If you could give advice to your younger self about your orgasm (or your body), what would it be?

Only do what your body wants. Do not let yourself be peer-pressured into pleasing others just to be liked or to conform to other people's ideas or standards.

If your orgasm had a voice, what would it say to you about the piece you wrote for this book?

It would say that it's glad I was able to reclaim my voice and be the director and producer of my life.

Anything else?

Your orgasm is yours and only yours. You need only yourself to have one, but it is fun to have someone to share it with.

Twelve

Reclamation of My Orgasm

by Cindy Anne

From my teenage years until recently, my orgasm was a one-note wonder.

At 48 my orgasm changed; it became a melody, a symphony of pleasure, of delight, of euphoria.

How did this happen, you might ask. Can it happen for me, you may wonder.

My honest answer is, I do not know. I can tell you the story of when my orgasm changed and the significant emotional event that happened before the changes. The story is not a story I enjoy sharing, but for you and your orgasm I will share.

My father began molesting me when I was twelve until about sixteen. I did the right thing when it first happened by telling my mother. I told her that when she sent me to my father's house he would fondle me. She asked me what I was wearing and what I had done to provoke this interest. I was twelve years old, in bed, asleep; I was unsure what I had done to draw attention to myself. These late night interactions, which were apparently my fault, were my first introduction to sex, as well as my awareness of myself in a sexual/sensual/horrified/scared/powerful/victim capacity. My first introduction to arousal was my father. I hated my life, I hated myself, I hated my ability to excite men without trying, yet it also felt amazing to have such power. Until this time, I had no idea I had this power!

I believed there was nothing I could do to stop my father, so I ran away. I lived on the streets of Seattle for several months before finally coming home to my mother's house. After that, I promptly got a boyfriend, got pregnant and lived happily ever after. Wouldn't it be nice if the story really ended like that? I lasted about ten years as a middle-class housewife to a local firefighter before falling apart and getting a divorce. My nightmares were haunting. My life was a fraud. And worse than any of this? I could never achieve orgasm without the image of my father in my mind.

I tried many ways to end this image but, at the final point of orgasm, there he was, fondling me to climax. I came to hate sex! I used it only as a way to keep men serving me. I avoided orgasm, the one-note explosion, as much as possible. If I could have sex and pleasure without orgasm it was great. If I had an orgasm my body would shut down afterward. I would pass out, feel the remorse and shame, wake up and pretend it was all grand. The orgasms felt good, but I hated the thoughts that filled my head. In my mind it seemed the best course of action to end these thoughts was to kill myself. I tried, but thankfully it did not work. However, I did spend several days in a psych ward and learned that I had something referred to as post-traumatic stress disorder (PTSD). I was in my twenties then. I did not tell anybody, including all of the doctors and therapists who tried to help me, about the orgasms and why I hated myself so very much.

I learned to live with this haunting for another 20 years; I no longer had a desire to kill myself. I went through years when I did not allow my father around me at all. I had complete breakdowns if he showed up at funerals or other major events.

Over time and with a lot of help, I forgave him. He himself has spent 25 years in recovery and has apologized for what he did to me. The apology does not change the facts. The apology did not change my orgasmic hauntings. The one thing that the apology did give me was permission to acknowledge, at least to myself, how being molested had affected me.

In 2013 I took a class in NYC. I had flown four hours, got little sleep, was in a different time zone and could not figure out how to find my favorite foods. All in all, I was absolutely spent. That is when it happened–when I was lonely, hungry and tired, I was pushed, and I had no way to edit my emotions. I had no strength to stop the gates from opening and releasing the flood.

I was sitting in my chair. One of my classmates insisted on going up on stage and telling her story—her story about how each man in her family had had his way with her sexually, and how she felt like she had never owned her own body.

I lost it.

I started to cry. I fell to the floor, curled up into a ball and started to hyperventilate. The words, "never owned my own body" knocked everything out of me. A group of women gathered around me. The facilitator asked if I was ok. In a dream-like state, I stood up. I asked for the microphone, and to the 250 women who sat before me I told the biggest, darkest, most shameful secret of my life.

"I can't orgasm without thinking of my father. I try, and he still shows up each time." With that I collapsed back to the floor and continued my sobbing.

I was quickly surrounded by the angels that were my classmates. They wrapped me in coats. They stroked my hair. One woman even got on the floor, held me in her arms and rocked me, whispering in my ear that I was safe.

This was truly a significant emotional event.

When I got home from New York I told my boyfriend, who later became my husband, all about what happened over the weekend. I felt very vulnerable as I shared this truth with my most intimate partner, the man who desired to bring me to orgasm and yet would now know the truth of that orgasm. He loved me anyway. He loved me from a place of truth and tenderness. Our lives changed from that moment on.

That was almost three years ago.

The first change I noticed after my weekend was that my body no longer became tense prior to orgasm. The next thing that happened, almost by magic, was that I realized my father was nowhere in my mind at the point of orgasm. With these two changes in my body I began to trust. I started to relax during sex. For the first time in my life, I was neither avoiding nor forcing orgasm. I began to surrender to the amazing way my body felt. From this relaxed state of being, my body has started to have long, rolling, expansive orgasms, usually multiple times. There are even points when I achieve orgasm without being touched. The look in my husband's eyes and his energy and love flowing to me is enough for my body to drop into a state of ecstatic orgasm.

By sharing my nightmare out loud, my shame and the voices that created that shame disappeared.

I tell my story in hopes that it helps somebody reclaim their orgasm as I was able to reclaim mine.

About the Author
Cindy Anne
www.agirlsroom.com

If your orgasm had a voice, what would it say to you about the piece you wrote for this book?

My orgasm has become the universal flow that moves through all beings.

Through orgasm my soul now bursts into everything and nothing all at once. It then comes back, back to the center of the I AM that I am... that is the multitude of explosions that today are my orgasms.

THIRTEEN
THIS WILD RISE
by Rebecca Holt

Weaving Mantra
Winds of the South, West, North, and East
Take this weaving of my soul
Allow the golden honey of these breathing words and this
holy sound current
To ride on the beloved wings of angels,
as it spins the highest love for the heart, body and soul of
the world
Let it be
a breathing, a cradling prayer, a living love sonnet
For all
That they may be reminded of the Deep Low Hum,
The deep, rich, nurturing current of creative life force
that flows in, through and beneath us all
We are being poured into grace and space
Nature's breath
and nurtured awning
In the name of the Divine, of God, the Weavers,
of Pachamama, of the Infinite
I'm declaring
Thank you thank you thank you
Blessed be and blessed we
—Rebecca Holt

Several years ago I synchronistically discovered an online prayer written by a very moving woman, who is a Sardinian sea silk weaver and sea singer. She is one of the oldest of her generation who still weaves and sings and teaches others the arts of her lineage. She sings her ancient traditional healing songs to the sea, and then listens deeply for the spaces that are open to gifting. She then dives down deep into the depths of the Mediterranean sea to gather the sacred bivalve mollusc shells in order to spin and weave golden byssus sea silk thread from their inner shell, and then returns the shells to the sea, to breathe once again the current of the deep healing waters. When I uttered the words of her prayer, it was as if honeycombs had been spun through my cells. The golden honey nectar of her holy soul calling prayer continues to flow through my bones. Her words inspired me to listen deeply for the unfolding of my own breathing mantra.

It is my prayer that my mantra above and my breathing words invoke in you a reclaiming, a knowing, a soul's calling back to the holy art of loving yourself in the widest and wildest of ways.

People shrink when they hear me say
People shriek when they hear me say
The weight of the world is on
Women's weight is on the world
The weight of the world is on the girls

Shrinking to see her light
being brings up the fright
breathing the old tangled night

Broken
coerced
unseen
outside of her body she flies
can you hear her silent cries

In the magical whispers of dreamtime
you can hear her softly chime
> **my firelight still shines**
> **in the center of me**
> **I remember that way once**
> **the lure of my heart**
> **Its grand paying attention**
> **listening into the cells**
> **through the layers**
> **I would swim**
> **finding the rhythms**
> **beneath my skin**

Be with all of this beautiful noise
let it lilt the body
the way the light and wind
pray on the meadow

Lovingly
knowingly
informing the soul
in its rocking

See how she rises up
firing her brilliance
into the mystery

The old way
calls her name
from time to time
yet she is already dancing
with the stars

We are gathering here
humming the notes of tides
weaving the symphonies of SHE

The old weight
has fashioned grooves for grace
breathing in feather-like freedom
The ancient witness
is singing its way back
into her bones

She is leaping now
into the waves
of this new hymn
©Rebecca Holt

I am singing over the bones of those who wish to connect to what I call the Deep Low Hum...that great song, that ancient current that flows in, through, above and beneath all of us. The Oran Mor, the Sea Melody, the great song at the center of our force of creation. The seed of unexpressed creative essence that is behind our breath, behind our voice, behind our heart. The pulse of pure, raw, creative consciousness that leads us to our own becoming. This pulse has a sound, a vibration, a creative force that leads us home to our own rising.

> **When we rise from our own power and use our soul voice**
> **to stand up and to be counted, in the truest, most beautiful**
> **expression of who we are. The world joins us in our symphony!**
> **©Rebecca Holt**

> **Be spun**
> **as you embark on the journey of this one love**
> **this path of rising**
> **Rising in love with your own undying heart**
> **Rising in love with the skin you are in**
> **Rising into your own pleasure**
> **your own nurture**
> **your own rapture**

> **I am feeling moved to speak to you in watery ways**
> **ways that soften, move and shape, and soothe**
> **The ways of sound and mantra, sacred ritual, metaphor and poetry**
> **have become my living, breathing well of transformation**

My yoga training teacher and dear soul sister, Corena Hammer, shared this Sanskrit mantra with us in yoga training one day…

HARI OM TAT SAT TU: TO THINE OWN SELF BE TRUE

As we all joined in the mantra in unison, the medicine of these heart-warming Sanskrit words melted into my cells, engraving their meaning into my breath. This mantra was a seed planted in me that day of remembering to always listen to my own inner whisperings of knowing and deepest heart desires to always have my own back. Ever honoring and bowing to the very center of my own true nature.

I have been a witness to many people's greatest gifts and soul callings unfolding through some of their most extremely difficult and traumatic experiences.

> When we are willing to move through the fear
> to thaw out the frozen
> to allow the old stories to die to the majesty of the unknown
> Our bones begin to breathe in the new stories
> to allow new stones and growth
> Our own inner wild creative life force finds its way back
> to the natural rhythm of the deep low hum…that great sea melody,
> the deep water current that lies in, through, above and beneath us all.

We can then embark on **THIS WILD RISE**, heart first!

CHANT YOUR HONEY FROM THE ROOFTOPS
[1]

Sing
Someone will find you
Your soul will pour itself into the ashes
Milling with ancient tides

Sand blast the way that wants to be paved through you
Guile is not your friend
Quietly mark your path
Showing signs to those who need the light
Their feet being guided as their eyes cannot yet see

Moving through layers of space
Feeling the ease
Sensing its grace
Colors begin to rush forth
Splashes of reddish purple and blue
I this you
This vibrant palette of creation
Aho Mitakuve Ovasin
Now bursting
with the symphony of "All My Relations"
  ©Rebecca Holt
  "Sing, sing a song, Sing out loud, sing out strong. Don't worry
  that it's not good enough for anyone else to hear, just sing, sing a
  song." (lyrics by Joe Raposo)

I can feel the avocado green, raised-patterned carpet between my toes and the dark 70s stained fireplace stone that had become the stage for my daily singing and dancing performance for my family. As a child, this was my favorite spot in the very center of my universe where I felt safe to sing out and to share the song of my heart, no matter its imperfections.

  It was in these magical moments that I could feel
  the music breathing me through my life. Music
  has always been a bridge, a place to plant my feet
  when finding my way...a healing balm for my heart
  and soul. Music literally reveals the truest expression
  of me. It sings me home to my own true nature.

From the time I was very young I loved anything to do with music, singing, sound, rhythm and dance... all of the avenues that assisted me to express the music breathing inside of me. Because of my early childhood traumatic experiences, I definitely had several parts of my soul that decided it was safer to take the exit door and go on an early vacation. These soul parts never left me, they moved up and outside the body to a place that felt safer... truly, to protect me. Through my shamanic energy medicine initiation and training with Alberto Villoldo's The Four Winds Healing Light Body School, I was given the gift and support to allow these parts to come back. These inner littles were greeted with gentle compassion, grace and healing medicine in order to integrate and resonate once again with my true heart and soul.

I have realized over time that I went unconscious during my early childhood abuse. These experiences happened over several years between the ages of three and six. I had symptoms throughout my life of fainting and always wondering if something had happened to me. Through the years, I repeatedly asked my mom if she could remember anything. Deep down I always knew, my body knew, my heart knew, my cells knew, my soul knew. The memories were deeply locked away and would come out in my dreams at times as night terrors. I remember for several years fleeing my bed and running to my parent's room for refuge after seeing dark figures in my room at night, or hearing dark noises. I remember a Dracula and a shark that I felt dwelt in the space between the wall and my bed. I was horrified to close my eyes at night. I was born bow-legged and had a pair of special shoes with braces around my legs and feet and bars across my toes that I had to wear to bed for 6-8 months. During this time I would still crawl to my parent's room at night on most nights... and I can still remember the sound of the shoes dragging across the floor. It was always a sigh of relief when I would make it to the safe refuge of their bedroom. My heart could breathe, my body could let go of the holding... the tight holding that I don't think I let go of until my late twenties.

Around the age of twenty-five, some of my more cognitive vibrant memories began to emerge while working with a therapist and body worker. One night I went over to a relative's house to visit and sleep over. Randomly the man who had abused me, was visiting my relative's home. I went to bed that night and upon waking the next morning, it was as if I had been riding a horse for two years as hard as I could. My entire groin area was exhausted and I could feel my entire genital area weeping from its core. My body was obviously letting me know…this tightening, this holding was to protect me and was reeling from the shock that was lingering and stuck throughout my body. This tight holding has now released, relaxed and through breath, movement, poetry, sound, has become my inner truth that holds me together… that sustains me. The quiet anxious, tight place of holding was the catalyst that has led me to this inner place of still, solace, divine holding.

THE DEEP LOW HUM
[2]

Our soul songs
Outside of time
Dancing in rhyme
Silent earth prayers
Peeling the layers
Weaving through sunset
Their fiery tones
Wild and wide
Bursting hearts open
Refining the hues
Of our becoming
©Rebecca Holt

I have known that this sound, this current of creative healing song was simmering inside of me all of my life. I call this deep holy frequency of creative life force the Deep Low Hum. This is the current that I hear in and through everything. When I am doing my work I can hear this deep low hum as it slowly cradles us home. Going through the extremely difficult life and body numbing experiences of childhood trauma, where my own voice was shut down, literally frozen in time, where I was not able to stand up for myself, I have connected to my own medicine of sacred Sound Weaving and medicine poetry in every cell of my being.

I was born to sing, to bring sound and authentic voice to that which has been cut off, shut down...to allow freedom to pour literally through our soul voice. I believe that we are all born with a destiny that lies within us and mine is to "sing soul over the bones," as Dr. Clarissa Pinkola Este so eloquently puts it.

I weave sacred sound and poetry medicine to assist those who may have gone through childhood trauma where their inner littles were not free to speak out. To sing the song of the soul over the bones, that other dear ones can find their own deepest heart connection, their own divine creative expression. Also, for those in this world who are currently suffering from the life numbing experience of abuse, where the true nature of the soul has been frozen in time.

Through my sacred sound weaving, chanting and medicine poetry, it is my intention to bring true cell bursting joy, soul flight and freedom, and authentic expression to the shut down voices on this planet!!

What started out as dread in these bones
The heavy voices
have turned into choices

I spent a half-life trying to peel off this suit
then one day I realized
the very skin I was in
was my vehicle to freedom

Offer it up
a prayer to the wildest skies
nothing to do with size

Thus little
her voice was cut off shut down
and cries could be heard for miles at night
the crippling of fright
the creatures lingering
in the space between the crevice of the wall and the bed
this dread

It was in the red desert
she unleashed these cries
and their size
the self loathing
became lifetimes of holding

The weavers
The women
They came in droves
to relinquish her woes
unwinding her early experience of touch and of breath
Releasing the grips of death
bringing on the thaw
what was frozen in her jaw

Awakening her voice
the ancients poured through
her throat found the sound
coming up through her feet
from the ground
The wild dance of innocence restored
her truest heart no longer ignored

We are the sum of all our experience
and then not
we are all we got

It's time dear heart to shine
you don't have one more minute
to live through the old stories
frozen in time
They haunt and taunt
They promote the hiding

This life is calling you to a new song
to breathe new life into these bones
the new story of home
of lightness
of flight
These wings
will take you to the valley of kings

It's time to soar
Can you feel her
This wild rise
©Rebecca Holt

Since my early teens, I longed for and chased balanced health, searching for healing and the place of deep connection from the exterior world outside of me via almost every therapeutic avenue possible, from traditional cognitive therapy, psychotherapy, many modalities of energy release work, soul work, EMDR, EFT, birth transition work, NLP, holotropic breath work, to Native American ceremonies, shamanic energy work, workshops out in nature, yoga, energy work in the water, and sound therapy, etc. Although I was infinitely grateful for all of the transformational aspects of this healing work, as each piece had brought me to a deeper place of soul and body awareness and to an ancient modality and language of healing that I was called to remember, I was still searching with a scattered, longing anxious, unseen, unheard, unleashed little one's voice inside of me.

DESERT ON THE BODY
[3]

About six years ago, I discovered my wounded "inner little one" in the healing red desert of Southern Utah, a dear medicine place I like to call The Red Ocean, in a sweat lodge journey ceremony and literally brought her back to life. After going inward, and deeply listening to the wisdom of the healing land of the desert, to the whispering of the holy spirit, to my own higher self and deep inner knowing, and into this great melody…the current that flows in, through, above and below all of us, the heart beat of the earth that pulses through our bones. I breathed and sang soul over my own bones as we finished the lodge with all of our own healing sounds. My desert brother and teacher always call this last round of the lodge, "the spirit round." In this place in the middle of the desert, I was able finally to truly let go of the tight holding, to sit still and breathe in the sounds of my soul.

> **To sit is not to wait**
> **To hold does not distill the grate**
> **Wild spaces in between**
> **The moments go unseen**
> **Feel them**
> **Reveal them**
> **Unseal them**
> **Take note**
> **Take heed**
> **No haste**
> **No waste**
> **A taste**
> **A Brush with death**
> **My breath**
> **Unseeing the seen**
> **Moments green**
> **Voices**
> **unfolding choices**
> **Mind to matter**
> **Unveil the chatter**
> **Wild wild child**
> **She danced**
> **While you glanced**
> **At all the scary places**
> **She jumped into hairy spaces**
> **Cob webs cleared out**
> **Her clout**

Was fear
She knew
She always knew
And flew
Crying saved her
Dying made her
View the unseen
Stacking not packing
No grasping
Coming up for air
These words are signs
Unwind them
Or bind them
Shadows find them
Looking glass
Wardrobe's closet
Your magic
Tell it
Shout it
From the rooftops
You melt
©Rebecca Holt

I believe in life we are not given experiences that we cannot handle. I believe that I was called to teach, to heal and to sing out with the healing and creativity that breathes and weaves through

going deep deep down into the dark place of shadow
deeply listening
allowing the thaw
the letting go
the sloughing off
the death and grieving
then from that empty place our soul begins to slowly find its more grounded footing one step at a time.

We can resonate one *songline at a time more closely to the natural rhythm of our own true nature.

DARK EARTH PRAYERS
[4]

> **Moments pour in**
> **Experience weaving her silk layers**
> **Like dark earth prayers**
> **Echoes of story gently lifted**
> **Deeply rooted core restored**
> **As history's dust is sifted**
> **Senses heightened**
> **Voices streaming**
> **Fields of joyful stillness dreaming**
> **—Rebecca Holt**

Through many teachings in my life and instilling of beliefs through religion, in school, in as many places as I can remember, I was taught that the dark equaled evil or harmful places or energy. And because of my early childhood trauma, I lived through those years of night terrors where I abhorred the darkness. In my later years through my healing experiences and in the desert sweat lodge especially, I embraced the deep dark, womblike place of my own heart and the inside of my own skin, of feeling my breath and body comforted against the warm deep earth, seeing and feeling the embracing moon and the stars outside the lodge cradling all of us through the depths of the sweet healing darkness of the magical night.

The poetry medicine of Rainer Maria Rilke and David Whyte in their poems about the deep earth, holding, healing love in the womblike dark, has been a healing elixir for me in reshaping and reclaiming my love of the dark. We all came into this world for nine months sleeping, and swaying, and eating and being nurtured in the heart beat of the deepest darkest place of the womb. Rilke's poetry continues to assist me to unravel and understand the deep holiness of this loving, womblike inner contemplative landscape of the dark.

...no matter how deeply I go down into myself
my God is dark, and like a webbing
made of a hundred roots that drink in silence.
I know that my trunk rose from his warmth,
but that's all,
because my branches hardly move at all
near the ground, and just wave a little in the wind.
—Rainer Maria Rilke

Diving down into these deep, dark caverns enabled me to shed light on all the cracks that I thought were walls. I discovered the beauty and mystery in the idea that there are always shades and crevices of light inside the shadow.

As I continued to dig, to listen to those deep guttural sounds of release and of grief, to allow the digestion and death of the old experiences and the old stories, I was then slowly able to cultivate, to nurture and to reclaim those dear soul parts that lay dormant and the masked facets of my soul.

Discord
What is the center of this sound
The moon has carried you in with the tide
Throwing the compass out
This wild ride

The weight of these dark notes unravels my heart
every facet resonating with the darkest art
the dark here refers to the underbelly of the soul

The pieces that go
Unsung
Unnoticed
Untold

Listen in the stillness
now sit here for a few
your tired skin may remain here
while shedding this view
Devour the most unknown knowing you know
the ONE that moves you gently back into the
   flow

Be with these notes deep inside of your bones
with the syllables of your truth
reweaving your own
Prayers into the sound
Now breaking highest ground
©Rebecca Holt

The earth inside of me was transformed from a red/black barren desert to a green, blue, deeply moving, breathing, watering place of peace, breath, love, discovery and creation. I found the deepest place of breathing inside of me. The place of my own heart and soul, my own inner music... heartbeat and rhythm that could now meet up and dance with the heartbeat of the earth. When I lose sight and sound and a sense of this place now, I quickly go outside, up into the mountains, to the ocean, to my favorite tree, to the river, to the desert... out into nature, and I make the sounds that bring me back to this place of my own voice... my soul voice that connects with those of the ancient waters, of the ancient ones who have come to connect and to sing the soul and water songs of joy and love and deep intimacy over the bones. The Deep Low Hum that cradles us in all moments.

WILDLY PLANTED
[5]

Recipes for wildness
Read your favorite poems in the moonlight
Dance when no one is watching
Dance when everyone is watching
Recite the names of god and grace in every voice, prayer, tongue that
pours out of you

Submerge your feet in the earth
let them feel the deep holding
The sustenance for miracles
Listen to the trees and mountains
they whisper the ancient stories of the ancestors
they sing lullabies to the sinking heart and lull the sacred body to
alignment
The source of the I am that I am
Lies greatly within this holy practice
    ©Rebecca Holt

From the earliest time I can remember, I was obsessed with all things with
a harmony and rhythm. I loved drums and string instruments. I soon
learned that I had a natural love for songs that had many harmonies and
different parts. I remember sitting on the church bench with my mom and
sisters at the age where I discovered my natural love for harmony and my
natural ability to hear all of the parts of each song and hold the harmonies
while others sang around me. I remember feeling my heart welling up
every Sunday as I sang the hymns and felt the brilliant light that soared
through the music.

    Throughout my childhood I spent countless hours in my room
listening to music and picking out the multiple harmonies and intricate
tones. Music was a friend, a heartful companion to me in the loneliness.
The lyrics I shared above about singing your own song, no matter if it is
not good enough, pour into my heart now whenever I move to judge
myself in any way or when I feel critical of my own sound or music. They
have become a personal mantra for me to this day reminding me that

sound is all about expression of my own personal note on this earth, my own frequency of home. The weaving sound is not about a performance, it is truly about sharing our unique signature, our own expression of love and brilliance with the world.

These were the seeds planted in my childhood that pulled me toward the world of healing sound and falling deeply in love with the holiness of our own wild and precious lives.

Later in my life, I melted into this love affair with words, language, poetry and their power to create through cultivating these seeds. My mom read us poetry and fairy tales and stories throughout our growing up years; she always had an appreciation for the arts and music and instilled that love in all of us. I remember her reading the words and the poems moved through me like songs. I realize now that poetry and music moved in and through my bones as medicine even back then. I think that my body was not yet ready to receive the fullness of these gifts.

Words and sound come into me
Like desert on the body
Arise and fall
In between moments recall

Humming on the wind
Oozing through my skin
Like tasting silky soft lips
As they open to my tongue
With a river's current
They are wild and new
Moving my heart and mind
With each moment's hue

My throat finds the sound
Like quiet whisperings of juniper
Landing on red sifted chocolate ground
Moving in and out of my breath
Like the beat of my drum

Infinite windows of rapture
Prisms of freedom

Stillness and chaos
Rhymes move into being
Shaping every moment they touch
Like a breeze, a kiss, a wave, a babies laugh

I welcome them home
To sit in the warm sun and sip them a while
Sun sets and the words
join the moon dust
Dissolving into stars
once again
Like nights ocean
Mystery combining
©Rebecca Holt

My dearest teacher and soul friend Trina West says, "in breathing I touch my own divinity." All of our words, songs, stories, prayers poetry and mantra begin with the breath. We are all living breathing poetry. I feel like the medicine of poetry is similar to that of prayer. It encompasses our deepest words emerge from the breathing heart of our soul, then are written, and shared or uttered out loud for the purpose of invoking.

All of life is a prayer of poetry to me. I can feel the words and sound that make up this poem of life that we are all living in. We are always revising, we are always rewriting, renewing, reclaiming. Just like the lines of a poem are under constant revision, we are ever transforming as beings in each moment, in each breath. We are the architects of our lives, of our experience, of how we perceive and learn and grow from our experiences. We are moving poems of living breathing creation.

We are by nature
a living breathing prayer
pulsating the wind
the sheets of our breath

Divine architecture
penetrating the veils of this wave
weaving its way
into the grooves
of the silent roots
fashioning the very center
of our dance with creation

Gliding melodiously
along the corridors of this lilt
we are birthing
the breathing silhouettes
of our soul's calling
©Rebecca Holt

With each breath I can empty out the chatter of my busy thoughts, which allows stillness and space. Into this space I am pouring laughter, love, sunshine, creativity, and joy!

For me poetry is getting in touch with the wild, joyous, beautiful, rapturous, creative expression inside of me and at the center of my own true nature. Nature brings me right back to my very center, that place of the wild, cradling feminine.

Poems are a timeless weightless balm
that beckons the mind, body and soul inward
To draw upon the tranquil sea
Find your favorite poems
Visit them often
©Rebecca Holt

When the timing was right in my adult life, the frequency of the words and weaving sounds began pouring back, beckoning me inward, to visit the darkness, the shadow, to sit still within this place and breath in soul… to breath health, balance, beauty, freedom, and heart burning love into the cracks and spaces and moving the blockages from the early trauma that otherwise would have rendered me frozen for good. When I was in my early twenties I will never forget my mom coming into my sister's bedroom and asking us all to lie down. She turned on an audio recording of David Whyte, one of my most favorite transformational poets of our time and she played the audio version of his poem, *The Opening of Eyes*.

I remember hearing the cadence of his voice repeating the last line of that poem where he talks about Moses in the desert and his experience of pure holy astonishment of being present and grounded in surrender. The words of this poem and the medicine of David Whyte's voice, were like a hand that reached into the cement in my chest, into the sedentary confinement of the frozen stories, and pulled me out of the quick sand out of my own deeply introverted, deeply stuck and frozen story... his words brought the breath... the fire... the water... the earth to all of my cells. I was infinitely changed.

WORDS THAT BREATHE
[6]

> **Spoken words create worlds**
> **Our truth lives deep down in our soles**
> **Breathe from there**
> **©Rebecca Holt**

Our words are pockets of frequency that literally create what we are speaking. I have learned through my personal devotional practice with Sanskrit mantra meditation, of the power of the spoken word to create momentum and the power of speaking in the direction we are moving. Our words and sound frequency are powerful tools for creation and transformation. When used with deep intention they can create worlds.

As I have been flowing going back through time and the experiences that have shaped and honed both my earlier escape from and my later embodiment of the skin that I am in, and the breathing of life down deep in my own bones, I notice that music and words have so lovingly carried me through all of the tides and seasons of my life. I was born with music pouring through my veins and the poetry found me mysteriously and divinely at precisely the right time. One of many "god moments" in my life, I feel like it was a sense of remembering a very ancient part of me that has always been there. This awareness and love affair with music, sound and medicine poetry catapulted me to leap into my work of singing the true song of the soul over the bones. My grandpa was an author and writer and he wrote several books of poetry. I remember him sharing poems with all of us gathered round. His words enchanted me, they took me away to the "chimney that stands alone" out in the desert landscape. He was a peaceful, introverted man of grand inner stature... a true cowboy at heart; he raised Arabian horses and had a passion for them. He also loved to plant and cultivate trees and the land; a gardening farmer of sorts. In quiet sunny summertime spaces, I feel his love of landscape, of poetry, and of words sitting on the air just above me... inspiring me to continue to free and share my own soul voice, so that others can free their own!

Late one night in my meditation I was asking the divine for a name that could encompass my soul work of sacred Sound Weaving and medicine poetry. I went to bed and woke up very early in the morning with my guides speaking these words directly into my right ear...

"WORDS THAT BREATHE"

Right then this name that has called my work into being became the wave of energy that flows through all of my poetry and sound-weaving expression.

**Our soul songs, the frequency of our own true nature,
our chants, our hums, our songs, our words
the tides of our lives
are a form of poetry
that is literally breathing
us home.
©Rebecca Holt**

FREE YOUR MIND
[7]

Bark
Bark at the thing that quiets you
Challenge the fear of embarrassment
It is only a moment
where the little one hid
from the terror of laughing

The shunning of those
who didn't know their own sunshine

She came here
To jump into those spaces
The wide open canyons
Where the very bright pieces of the soul
Will sing

She weaves courage and power
with her breath
The kind of knowing
that wakes up the dead

This rebirth can sting with the first breath
And then the second
is a falling into the nature of this golden hue
Running through the veins
Calling us to shine
©Rebecca Holt

I believe that we all have our own unique sound, our own note of expression to breathe out into the world. When I began to do healing sound I realized that the key for me was unlocking or releasing the spirit or soul to soar. I was asking one day of my higher self what my passion was for this work and the word FREEDOM came to me. Freedom has so many different meanings for all of us.

When thinking of the deepest sense of freedom, I am reminded of one of my most favorite movies of all time, *Braveheart*. In the last scene he is lying on the execution table being asked to cry for mercy in order for his life to be spared. This scene is forever engraved in my consciousness.

There is sublime silence in the overlooking crowd for a few moments…

You can truly hear a pin drop.

Then there are the forlorn faces… of women, and children

the broken faces of his soul brothers with their hearts being ripped out

the haunting faces of those cheering the executioner on

The agony and the exhaustion in so many and the essence of an ultimate giving up in the energy of the crowd.

And then through the pool of silence

William Wallace belts out with undying, powerful, life-wrenching creative life force, the word…

"FREEEEEEEDOM!"

As I originally recalled this scene, and whenever I call it back up now, I can feel the tears welling up in me. I can feel the power that our expression has to set us free as it freed William Wallace from his suffering.

My early childhood trauma silenced my voice and bound up the little girl in me who wanted to sing out. Through these extremely difficult experiences I learned of the power of unleashing my own voice… of being able to sing out and stand up in the beauty and vibration of my own true soul.

I am gathering those who wish to connect to that unstruck sound, the "anahata nada," the seed of unexpressed creative essence that is behind our breath, behind our voice, behind our heart… the pulse of pure, raw, creative consciousness that leads us to our own becoming. This pulse has a sound, a vibration, a creative force that leads us home to ourselves and to our own rising.

When we rise from our own power and use our voice to stand up
and to be counted, in the truest, most beautiful expression of who we are
The world joins our symphony
     ©Rebecca Holt

You will find now the medicine that has been part of my daily cultivation practice of the love affair with this life of mine, with this body, mind, heart and soul I was born with. My poetry remedy below for all those circular thoughts that don't align with whole body loving, soul-igniting, cell-kissing, bone-dancing, rhythmic love infusion that lights a fire under our truest nature reminding us to shine.

> This one percent of body image heroin
> is like a water fall of pressure
> It feeds a fire
> that never goes out
> The fuel gets low
> and the weight fills up the kettle
>
> Black is the color of sludgy soot
> It seeps into the mind
> and all through the cells
> This is not the sunshine I was here to paint
> The shadows can lurk
> as if they were rainbows
> Their language has a disguise
> A mask that blinds
> What is the medicine?
> I plead
> The breath, prayer and mantra
> believe it or not
> are some of the finest ways
> for bailing yourself out of quicksand
> This mire was not meant
> A lifetime of housing the ox

Visualize the ocean
The tides
The colors
The frequency of waves

This is the flow
that fills the pores with home
The golden elixir of breath and light
sounds that arouse the senses
to their deepest place of knowing

Sink into this new well
one that allows the dark
to be your solace and your solstice
not a vice for drowning

Drink this golden nectar
Peaks will begin to grow
in your soul

The summit is endless
you are already soaring
in the mountain's highest ways
©Rebecca Holt

Creating sacred space, ritual, and ceremony, and being extremely present in my own moments of solitude are crucial tools that allow me to connect to my own inner wisdom and my own deepest heart desires. When things feel scattered and chaotic or out of sync, when I feel the absence of flow, or when I feel like I've lost my magic, I remember the place of the mythic: sound, storytelling, dance, poetry, sacred ceremony and also immersing myself in the ocean the mountains and laying under trees. I find my way back to the Deep Low Hum, my connection to the divine source of all that is, where all of life is a poem. Maryanne Williamson talks about the power of altars for transformation. That when we place things on the altar they are altered and cannot help but be transformed.

I am deeply grateful for the gift of sacred weaving sound and poetry medicine in my life, and for their reaching in and waking me from the deep frozen sleep of my early childhood trauma. My dear teacher, Trina West, told me once, "our bones hold our stories." Sound Weaving and breathing medicine poetry have unraveled, cleared out, and assisted in the peeling off of the old layers allowing them to die, supporting me to plant new seeds for the return to and reclaiming of my own true nature.

It is my prayer, my mantra, my grandest invocation...
That you will rise into the beauty of the skin you are in
That you will begin this dance with the golden honey inside of
your cells today

What New Way Wants to Rise Up in You?

What new way wants to rise up in you
what tiny bud
is stretching
out of the sacred ground

The ashes
have cleared the ground
for your desire
quickening the very seeds of devotion

Moving your heart in waves
You can hear the whispering
of canyons
red ocean tides
of inner miles

Uttering
> **breathe yourself onto this sacred road**
> **the way**
> **you have always known**
> **is holding your own**
> **Spring forth**
> **to the season of your combining**

This love
these sounds
are calling you
to the center of your own hearth

Breathe them
Speak them
Sing them
Join in your own symphony

Enter the canyons within your bones
Explore all of the low lands
Reclaim your own inner fire

Shout from the rooftops
this moment
and the next
and the next are
bringing you home
©Rebecca Holt

I am deeply moved and grateful to the divine, to The Weavers, to our ancestors and guides and to Pachamama. They are literally cradling us in all moments.

With warm golden honey prana mama earth elixir and blue ocean weaving sounds and love.

—Rebecca

About the Author
Rebecca Holt
www.wordsthatbreathe.com
Instagram: @wordsthatbreathe

What did you want to be when you were eight years old?

A singer, songwriter, sunshine spreader, prism lover, dreamer.

If you could give advice to your younger self about your orgasm (or your body), what would it be?

I am blessed to share here in the breathing pages of this book some whisperings of inner wisdom and knowing with my younger self...my own precious inner little

> **"Courage dear heart"**
> be spun
> as you embark on the journey of this one love
> falling in love with your own pleasure... your own nurture... your own rapture
> feeling moved to speak to you in watery ways
> ways that soften, move and shape, and soothe
> the ways of sound and mantra, metaphor and poetry have become my living, breathing stories

Hari Om Tat Sat Tu: "To thine own self be true"

This small poem below is written by one of my favorite poets, Nayyirah Waheed, who has a gift with gentle yet life-invoking words that open a world inside of us toward more radical self-love, more self-nurture, and deeper self exploration. It supports my sentiment above of always being true to our own being in all ways.

I am mine
before I am ever anyone else's
—Nayyirah Waheed

Fall in love with your Own
Breathe life and sing wild flower melodies
to the layers inside of your bones
to this body that is home to your soul
The moonlight inside of your skin
will begin
igniting the fire
that burns through your life
invoke all of the golden honey nectar of your soul
this wild rise

If your orgasm had a voice, what would it say to you about the piece you wrote for this book?

In this moment as I listen deeply into the middle of this deep low hum
I am reminded of the beautiful, moving words of one of our dear heart-
drivers in Bali, Leroy...
"Everything we do is prayer."
There is a moment inside all of it
where your heart just bursts
and connects to everything
that is GOD

Anything else?

Ask, listen breathe
in all moments
you are held in the arms of wild, limitless, divine sacred love
grounded by the roots of the mother trees
held by the wings of hosts of angels
cradled by the sounds of the wind and water songs
singing through your own sails
nurtured by layers of sea skies and chime
serenaded by swooning moon songs
You are grounded in timelessness
breathe into the earth

all that weighs you down
gather up the warm milk and honey nectar
manna for the body and soul
golden honey prana mama earth elixir
drink in all of this astonishing light
allow it to ignite all of your cells
feel the place of home within your center
breathe and move from here
embody your bones
sink in to this frequency of home
with warm deep-rooted silken sounds of moonlit magic

—Rebecca Holt

FOURTEEN
50 SHADED POEMS
by Cassy Fry

The piece featured is from my book 50 Shaded Poems, a collection of blackout poetry made from Fifty Shades of Grey that transforms text from a problematic novel into poignant and playful poetry.

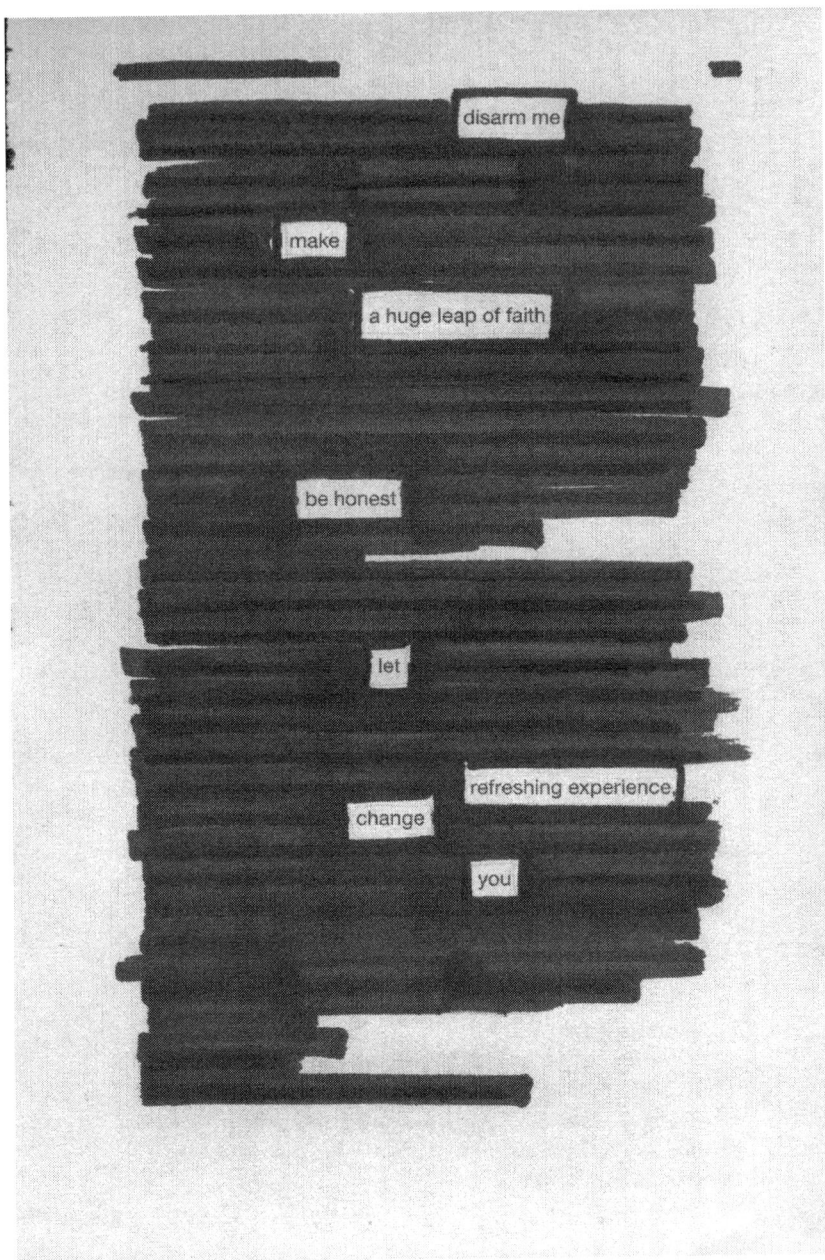

disarm me

make

a huge leap of faith

be honest

let

refreshing experience.

change

you

About the Author
Cassy Fry
www.cassyfry.com
Instagram: @CassyFry

What did you want to be when you were eight years old?

A gymnast—but I realised by the time I was ten that I was getting too old and should have already been in professional training, so then I did gymnastics just for the joy. Remembering how it felt to move my body like that makes me smile.

If you could give advice to your younger self about your orgasm (or your body), what would it be?

Do not feel guilty about feeling pleasure; your body has its own ideas and desires, and what makes you wet will often surprise you. You can step away from shame and enjoy yourself while still respecting yourself and your boundaries.

If your orgasm had a voice, what would it say to you about the piece you wrote for this book?

Thank you for recognising my beauty.

FIFTEEN
SEXUALITY AT ITS PEAK
by Leigh Hurst

I trusted the first male in my life to help me achieve orgasm. He was young, like me, and he convinced me that I could not get pregnant by him. Four months later I was pregnant. I was seventeen years old.

We married and spent the next twenty years together. During that time, I gave birth to two more children. When my kids were five, four and newborn, I went to school to earn a degree in psychology and another in social work while also studying gerontology and sex and aging.

I loved researching, learning about and discussing sexuality. The majority of humans engage in sex, but few like to talk about it or enhance their sex lives. I learned that most doctors are not even trained to help people age in their sexuality. I got halfway through my master's degree in gerontology before I went on sabbatical because sex and aging was not even a topic for discussion.

In my marriage, we had intercourse two to three times a week, but there was no kissing or intimacy. We told each other "I love you" out of habit. Even though I thought we had a healthy sex life, he cheated throughout our marriage with various women and prostitutes.

When my husband divorced me to marry someone else, I decided I was going to give myself five years of no men, no sex, no dating. Everyone thinks they need to find someone right away to complete them, but I wanted to discover who I was and what I wanted out of my life before I committed to someone else. I wanted to learn to love myself. I also chose not to put my children through different boyfriends, husbands or potential stepchildren that I saw in other post-divorce relationships.

I started attending yoga and reading many spiritual books. I was lucky to have an older man (79 years old) as my mentor, with whom I could talk about sexuality, finances, and my new journey. My youngest child nicknamed him "Tedward" and it has stuck through our relationship. Tedward was the first person to introduce me to the book *A Course in Miracles*. He taught me how much easier it is if your rent or mortgage is paid before the due date. We spent many hours building our friendship. He is the only person in my life with whom I could speak of sexuality so freely, and I in his. Any chance he got, he encouraged me to better myself as a person and develop my spiritual side.

Nearly five years later, I was an independent woman. I had paid off my car, got braces for both my daughters and bought my first home. As a woman I could feel myself growing into adulthood and a more mature way of living. At this time I still had not fallen in love with myself and did not feel quite worthy; there was still something missing in my life. I had not been introduced to my sensual side or had an awakening of any sort. It seems that I was still somewhat lost and had not connected to anything bigger than myself.

During my journey with Tedward I completed my master's degree in gerontology. He said it was really just another piece of very expensive paper that I did not need. He said I already had it in me as a person—all I needed to do was show it to the world. I completed almost half of that degree and felt frustrated that the studies were focused on so many theories but so little about sexuality and aging, so I stopped attending. I needed people who thought like me and saw sexuality as a way of life and not something to be ignored.

As chance would have it I was invited to a tantra event. At the time I had no idea what tantra was about. It seemed that it was lovers being connected to a source (God) and more connected with their sensuality. Tedward kept asking me why I felt I needed to attend this event, and I told him I really had no idea, but something inside me said I had to be there. My intuition told me that I needed to be at this event, even though I felt fear. Even though I had studied sexuality and talked about it, I was afraid—afraid that people would judge me. I was thin when I married my husband and never really stood completely naked in front of him. Now I had weight on me and felt body shame. I was also fearful that other students would be doing crazy things like having sex, and I feared that someone might want to have sex with me! I had been in a marriage of almost 20 years and then five years celibate. I felt like I had missed out on so many things that others had experienced in their young adult lives. It also seemed crazy at the time, because I never drove out of town alone, and here I was considering driving five hours!

I arrived the night before the workshop began, earlier than everybody else. Without the distraction of other people being there, unfortunately, I had time to feel my nervousness and trepidation. I started thinking about the terrible tantra stories I'd heard of group sex and everyone getting naked together. Tantra, however, is really about being connected to the Divine, or to God, and becoming one with your partner—sacred sexuality. I went to bed feeling alone and out of place. I didn't sleep much that night. I thought about going home.

The workshop began the next morning with the instructor introducing himself and spending a lot of time going through the boundaries and agreements for safety during the retreat. He emphasized that everybody was supported to say no to anybody, including him, and that none of us had to do anything we did not want to do. Everybody would be able to feel the level of involvement they wanted with each exercise presented. After the detailed welcome circle, we did yoga to warm up our bodies and then a couple hours of intuitive dancing.

This was an experiential course about tantra practices, and after the lunch break I was able to witness what can only be described as magic. I had once seen a video of someone performing what is called energetic full body orgasm and thought the person was full of shit. Yet here I was witnessing something that I could not even imagine was possible. The instructor, Alex, was waving his arms around above an assistant, and gradually her body started to come alive and vibrate, eventually cascading into what I later learned was a tantric full body orgasm. After the demonstration and Alex answering a bombardment of questions, it was now our turn to start giving and receiving these sessions to each other. I paired up with a lovely young woman, and we were instructed to share with each other how we felt and what our expectations were for the sessions and, of course, who was going to go first. We both realized we were a little nervous, and we both started to feel shame arising in our bodies. Alex had talked about how many of us were conditioned in our childhoods to hold sexual guilt and shame, so we were prepared for this. I was aghast; I had never been completely naked in front of anybody, yet here I was making a conscious choice to do what felt like jumping off a cliff. I was taking off my clothes in a room of 40+ strangers to receive one of these magical energy healing sessions. I was very much in my head, telling myself that other students were looking at me and judging me. Anxiety came over me, and I was crying uncontrollably. Alex rushed over to talk me through the story I was telling about myself. I shared with him that I was so afraid the student next to me was watching me. Alex had me take a deep breath and look over at the other student. The student was in total bliss, receiving energy work from his wife—I don't think he even realized he was still in the room. Sometimes our thoughts can get the best of us if we forget to practice mindfulness. I continued with my partner and experienced energy work for the first time in my life. It was wonderfully relaxing.

At the end of the day, we sat in a circle, sharing about our experiences and asking questions. I still felt like I didn't belong there. Everyone else seemed more experienced and open than me. After the session, people made plans for the evening. All I wanted to do was to go to my room and be by myself. As I fell asleep, I decided I would get up in the morning and go home.

The next morning I got up and started packing my suitcase. I phoned Tedward and he said, "What are you doing? You aren't coming home are you?"

I said, "I just can't do this."

"Don't come home! You are meant to be there!"

I said, "OK, OK," as I was zipping my suitcase. It was one of the few times I didn't intend to take his advice. My room was cleaned and packed, and I was ready to go. Now it was time to go find the organizers and Alex to let them know I was leaving. On the way I met Alex in a meadow, and I let him know I'd decided to leave. He calmly asked me if I felt like sharing why. I gave him my explanation; he nodded and listened intently.

He replied, "I get that it's out of your comfort zone," in a loving, warm, deep voice. Then he asked, "For how much of your life have you felt unworthy?" I'd never been asked such a direct question about this. I didn't know where it came from, but I just burst into tears right in front of him. He gently looked at me and said, "Go ahead, I'll be standing here waiting when you're done."

After the discussion with Alex, I realized I was at this workshop for a reason. It was going to change how I viewed relationships, but at the time I didn't realize it was going to completely change how I lived my life. I decided to be more open in the group, to let go of my fear and accept whatever was being brought to me. These lessons would all be valuable to me in my life.

The next morning Alex and I sat together by ourselves, eating breakfast. He gave me a little talk about relationships that morning. After spending twenty years in my last relationship, I really was searching for some kind of change. Alex said he had asked many women why they want to be in a relationship.

My first thoughts were because of the conditions we were raised in. The television shows we watched showed women in long-term marriages. I told Alex that this, however, does not work in our society any longer. Alex replied, "Leigh, some of the women I have asked shared that they wanted to be in a relationship because they want to have a baby, companionship and regular sex. They said, 'I want someone to talk to at the end of the day.' In the new paradigm for relationships, those are not reasons to be in relationships. Leigh, we can have all those things if we get more friends, if we buy a puppy or see a counselor for someone to talk to. We can get all those needs met by other people."

Alex finished up by sharing with me that what our sexual relationships give us, more than anything else, is a reflection. The reflection is everything inside us that is not loving, everything that we do not accept within ourselves. It gives us the opportunity to see that stuff more clearly, so we have the opportunity to heal those old wounds and to evolve beyond them.

I had been hearing people speak about sacred sexuality, but I told Alex I didn't understand what it was about. As we finished our breakfast and headed to class he said, "The new paradigm of sacred sexuality is about us taking self-responsibility and then being able to share intimately with each other. It's not about creating a power-over dynamic but a power-with dynamic, and that can only happen through self-responsibility and understanding that our relationships, especially our sexual relationships, are about reflection."

At that moment I realized that I was extremely sapiosexual (a person who is attracted to intelligence in others) and possibly a person who might want to explore having multiple open relationships. Breakfast was now over, and it was time to go begin the day's workshop. I had no idea what had happened to me in the last 24 hours, but I could feel a small shift happening.

As we all sat in the morning circle, we discussed how we had been feeling. After the talking circle, I decided I wanted to be paired up with a man for that day's exercises. I spoke with Mark, the fellow student I chose to work with, about boundaries for the sessions. I felt ok with him taking his clothes off. I made it clear I wouldn't be taking mine off, with which he agreed. As he got naked and lay on our area, I felt a sense of nervousness and unworthiness. Mark was a body worker, a massage therapist, and I was but a social worker.

As our time together began, I did what we had been learning and tried to move energy by waving my arms about, but I didn't really know what I was doing. Mark was starting to micromanage, telling me I wasn't doing things right. Alex saw what was happening and came over from behind me and gently whispered into my ear, "Do you want to be doing this?" I replied with yes. Then he said, "Maybe it's time for you to step into your

144

power." With that I felt a rush of energy up my spine. I felt my power. Mark was still trying to control the situation, and I was unaffected. I tapped into my intuition and started feeling energy moving through his body. For some reason I moved my thumb to the roof of his mouth as I had seen in a demonstration, and something magical happened. As surprising to him as it was to me, he had a full body orgasm without ejaculating. In that moment I found an answer to all I had been researching about sex and aging. People tend to believe sex is always about penetration and having ejaculations. During this time with Mark, witnessing him receive pleasure throughout his body without the need to have intercourse with me was a solution to all I had been studying about sex and aging. Just because we age and our genitals do not work the way they use to doesn't mean we need to stop having sex or intimacy. It means educating ourselves on how to create intimacy as we age. Neither of us could believe what had just happened.

Now it was time for the partners to switch places. As Mark got up he gently said, "It's up to you. You can leave your clothes on or take as much off as you like; I'm happy either way." I was relieved, as he reminded me of the retreat boundaries, which meant it was up to me to decide how far I would go. I lay down with my clothes on, and Mark started to move energy throughout my body. He also started asking me, "When did you start feeling so unworthy? When did you start telling yourself you weren't good enough, thin enough, attractive enough?" As he walked me through the story I'd been telling myself, I had one of the biggest cries of my life. I felt safe with it, though; I remembered the instructor saying that our vibration increases when our body releases emotional stress, and it's good to just go with it.

I felt so light and open after the release. I decided that I wanted to remove my clothes and see how that felt. Mark helped me remove my clothes. At first I felt anxiety and fear of being naked in front of a strange man. That thought left quickly, however, and I was ready to experience whatever Mark was going to offer me. He began again, moving energy through my body. If I have any type of cocktail or if the dentist gives me pain meds (I use only natural medicine now), I always feel it in my calves.

All of a sudden I felt my legs tingling. I shared this with Mark. I felt a wave wash over me as he laid his head on the part of my body I hated the most—my belly—and pressed on my pubic bone with his hand. I let go of everything, and my body vibrated, tingled and shook for what felt like forever. The instructor's voice brought me back to earth, saying we had twenty more minutes until lunch. Mark looked at me and started talking about me feeling shame about my body. I told him there's no time for that, my legs are tingling again! He said you want to do that again? Well, yeah! He started moving energy; I focused on my breathing, and this time it felt like my body lifted up and soared orgasmically across the room. I remember looking around and seeing people in the throes of energetic orgasm, with Alex standing in the middle, looking content and, I assume, feeling much happiness for us all.

After the session, even as I dressed, my body was still vibrating all over. I had never felt this before. I walked outside, and everything looked and felt completely different. The grass was greener, the sky was bluer, the air was fresher and there was more aliveness in my body. I could see Alex standing quietly in a meadow by himself enjoying the sunlight. I felt so much self-confidence going through me that I was drawn to go to him and express my gratitude. When I approached him he looked slightly puzzled, in a good way, and he gently said, "Sweetie, I get a sense you are ready to speak your truth."

"Yes, it is my truth for the first time in my life. My truth is I have been shut down sexually for some time. I haven't even kissed a man in twenty years, I haven't had sex in four and a half years, and I would like that to change. May we share in a kiss and have tantric sex?" He appeared open to that and suggested I take a little quiet time, and if I still wanted to after lunch, we could talk about it. I walked away feeling good about myself and confident that I had spoken my truth.

I sat down for lunch with the rest of the group, and they brought out the vegetarian food we'd had all week. I was over vegetarian food by then. My body was not used to vegetables and healthy food. I decided to go take some photos before class started. Taking photos has always been a meditation to me; it gave me time to reflect on my life and what I wanted and didn't want. I knew that I wasn't just caught up in the moment—what I had expressed to our teacher was my truth, and I wanted it to become my reality. I knew it was a possibility, because at the beginning of the retreat we had all discussed boundaries. Because this was a sexuality retreat for adults, it was OK to express our desires to other each other, including the instructor. We had all agreed upon that, so I didn't feel any shame about it. I went and found Alex, and we had a very lovely discussion about my motivations, and we decided to meet later that night.

When we met, we talked for a while about what I wanted from the experience. I decided I just wanted to kiss for a little while and see how that felt. To be that close to an individual's mouth and feel the rush of his breath from his lips before they touched mine was exhilarating. The quiet whispers and loving words that came out before the sweet kisses brought so much sensuality and excitement between us. The feeling of his mustache tickling my mouth and the smoothness of his lips were taking me to a state of ecstasy. It was such a relief after not kissing for twenty years to release this block I had around kissing.

After some time I decided I wanted to go further. I wanted to experience tantric sex with someone who could be very present, gentle and sensitive. We started breathing together and staring into each other's eyes. It felt like I had been missing this intimate connection my entire life.

I felt my vibration increasing very quickly and waves of pleasure rushed through my body. We stayed like that for some time, and then I decided that I wanted to go further once again; my body felt ready. We undressed and started having tantric sex. Alex gently placed his lingam inside my yoni, gazing into my eyes and connecting on a soul level that had my body feeling as if we were combining into one. At first I was moving all over the place; then Alex suggested I lie still a moment, and we slowly kissed. We started breathing together, and I could feel his lingam start to vibrate inside of me. It was intercourse like I had never experienced before. Instead of friction and moving in and out we were connected by our genitals, and the vibrations from Alex's lingam had my entire yoni vibrating with continuous, full-body energetic orgasms. I was experiencing so much pleasure, it was amazing!

Many times people are stuck in their heads, thinking during sex, or they get into a routine, or even feel an obligation to the other person. Alex, however, was very present, and he looked at me with so much love. I realized he did not have sex like any other man I had ever met. I didn't feel like a body anymore; I felt so connected to him in that moment of bliss. It felt like we had achieved unity of light and ecstasy. The thought ran through my mind, is this what complete happiness feels like? The love-making went on for some time. I could also feel his body vibrating like he was having energy orgasms as well. After what seemed like an eternity, my body felt complete in that moment, and I let him know. Afterwards, as I was leaving his room and walking down the hallway, one of the other women brushed passed me and said, "Honey, you're all aglow! Oh my goodness, did someone water your garden for you?" I had the biggest smile on my face. I headed outside, in total bliss.

At the end of the day, the group had a dance night to end the retreat. Never in my wildest imagination did I believe this event would change my life so much. Feeling like I had stepped into my identity as a powerful woman, I found Alex to tell him goodbye and thank you. He took me out to the middle of the dance floor, and we engaged in a passionate kiss in front of everyone! That sealed the experience for me, and I could move forward on my path with all my passion and power of being a wild, intelligent, beautiful, and compassionate woman helping others on their path. It was always there; I just needed some help to remove the old ideas and baggage I was carrying around with me.

About the Author
Leigh Hurst
www.awakeandaging.com

What did you want to be when you were eight years old?

At eight years old I wanted to be a teacher. I do believe I was a teacher in a previous life. I feel so lucky to be able to step into my teaching abilities and guide people on living a more conscious lifestyle and tapping into their sexuality.

If you could give advice to your younger self about your orgasm (or your body), what would it be?

If I could give my younger self advice about orgasm it would be to never stop learning how you can expand your pleasure. Let go of body shame and be present with your partner and allow your body to receive the tremendous amount of pleasure it was built for. Stop the self-talk in your mind and enjoy the experience.

To some people reading my story in this book it may seem strange being sexual at a retreat with the teacher, but I listened to my body and its needs and knew it was right for me. I never felt any pressure or manipulated. If anything, I felt I became a more enlightened, powerful being and that each woman should have an extraordinary experience such as this!

Once back home my life completely changed; I was no longer the woman that felt fear going to the retreat. I came home and made a completely different lifestyle for myself. I was always Catholic but gave up religion some time ago. I now feel extremely spiritual and connected to the divine, something bigger than myself. I feel more like a conscious being, sexy, alive and vibrant, being guided each day!

Some of the things that happened: giving up television, doing daily meditations, dancing when I feel stress coming on, becoming vegetarian sometimes vegan, giving up Diet Coke and chemical-filled foods and drinks, changing my style of music. I created my business, Awake & Aging, to teach and mentor people, not only about their sexuality and empowerment but also holistic wellness to create the greater good for their being.

The other fascinating thing that happened is I started dating younger men. I still work on my worthiness and how I look and feel. Younger men tell me they see me as their age, and as a goddess and an extraordinary woman. I also made the decision that committing to one person for the rest of my life is not for me. We are social creatures and have so much to offer each other, and I want to be able to feel free to make my own choices in my life. I feel truly awakened yet understand each day is a gift with new lessons for me to learn.

SIXTEEN

FIRE IN MY PUSSY
by Deborah Penner

My first memory of sexual sensation is of a stuffed bunny rabbit three feet tall that I used to put between my legs when I was nine as I went to bed because it Felt. So. Good. I would tell myself stories as I played with that bunny between my legs. That big stuffed bunny gave great head that promptly ended when I opened my mouth and told my mom. My fundamentalist missionary mama looked horrified.

"Stop it," she said.

She couldn't give me a reason. I did as I was told and stopped, but I wasn't totally convinced it was bad to feel that good.

Mom had already told me I couldn't square dance in PE.

"Good Christian girls don't dance," she said.

Fast forward to the year I graduated from high school. It was the end of 1973, and I was in the backseat of a car with a guy. It was our first date. We went out for dinner and a movie. I got him hard, so I figured I had to finish it. My thinking at the time was "Oh my god, I can't leave this man erect ... I don't want to be a tease!" I had no idea that penises get erect pretty much at the drop of a hat and that that physiological phenomenon occurs with or without me. So there I am in the backseat of the car having what I thought was my first sexual experience, and I couldn't understand the déjà vu of it. How could I feel as though I had been here before when this was clearly the first time someone's penis entered my body? I could not wrap my little missionary kid brain around that at all.

It turns out it wasn't my first sexual encounter. That happened at the beginning of first grade when I was raped in a classroom closet by a high school boy while another stood guard. I was six. He threatened to kill me if I told, and I believed him.

Dissociative amnesia is a six year-old's friend. The event was stored in an inaccessible part of my mind until the early 90s when my body started to remember and then again in 2013 when I consciously went after what was hidden in my unconscious with the intent of rewiring the skewed neurological connection around my experience of sex.

I had no conscious idea of any of that in the backseat of that yellow '57 Chevy station wagon. I felt as though I had no choice. Not because the man I was with—and would be with for the next four years—was coercive in any way. He was one of the most passive people I have ever known. The neurological response to sex established during the rape simply kicked in. Hard penis equals death threats.

He's the first person I felt an orgasm with. I remember the sensation clearly. It was a little like when my mom would stroke my back before I went to sleep sometimes, only a thousand times more intense. It started as fire in my pussy and moved down my legs and up my belly. It. Felt. So. Good.

I remember thinking, "Oh! That must be what it feels like." Nothing more. Just, "Oh that must be what an orgasm feels like. Okay, that feels good. I'd like more." I was very disconnected from the whole thing other than being on top, riding him when I experienced that burst of sensation, but there was no flipping passion with this man. It was like, I had an orgasm. That's fun! I'd like more; how do I do that? Very matter-of-fact. I certainly didn't share it with him. Not because it was scary. It simply didn't enter my mind to tell him.

Nobody had really taught me about sex. The extent of my sex education was the rape at six and my mother telling me at twelve how intercourse happened and that it was what married people did. My thought on that was, "Eww. Okay. What's the big deal?"

In the same way I knew there was more to the fundamentalist Christian story of the God that I was raised to fear. I knew in my bones there was more to this story of orgasm and female sexuality than I had been allowed (and had allowed myself) to know.

That first experience was the only time I remember climaxing with that man. Four years later, after I left him, I started researching sex (by allowing myself to have it with anyone I wanted) and reading everything I could get my hands on. I figured if I understood it, I might be able to experience it again. I committed to learning how to give myself pleasure and picked up where I left off with the stuffed bunny, devoting myself to my own orgasm.

There was a bit of militancy to the devotion. First, I couldn't depend on my partners to do it for me, and second, and more importantly, I didn't want to depend on them. It was so much easier to have control of it, and it felt so much safer. I could have sex, not worry about whether I climaxed and take care of it after he left, and men tend to fall asleep after sex, so it was not a difficult thing to pleasure myself to climax after they were done. And paradoxically, with each new encounter I was hoping to be taken over the edge of my resistance.

How you do one thing is how you do everything.

My relationship to my orgasm, to my pleasure, to my body was chaotic. Like my relationship with men. The neurological wiring of pleasure with fear and possible death was always running silently under the surface. After a while, it would kick in and sabotage any pleasure I experienced. I would push it away. I would push the one sharing it with me away.

The year of fucking dangerously ended abruptly when one of the men I engaged with decided he owned me. He broke into my apartment, read my journals and used the contents to control me. I was primed for that. I had just read *Looking for Mr. Goodbar*, a story of a woman who was doing as I was. She was killed by one her encounters. The fear that had been hovering just below my awareness moved smack dab into the center of it.

My open exploration of pleasure went underground, just as everything I loved in my childhood had. Underground was a place I knew and understood. Underground was a place I could control to a degree. It took twelve years, two husbands and a tiny end run into my old religion before I could allow myself to understand that alone might really be better. Every time I remarried or lived with a man, I had a sinking feeling in me, an "Oh no! Here I go again! Oh well, I'll get out of it eventually."

For a very long time, I walked around believing that the little and powerful bursts that I gave myself were the extent of my orgasm. That began to shift around the age of 42. I began to understand that everything is energy. My understanding of it was deeply enhanced by a long-distance relationship and technology. I felt him in the room during our play.

I opened to movement. Dance as prayer was a natural progression for me that began when *Sweat Your Prayers* by Gabrielle Roth nearly jumped off the shelf at me in the spring of 2000. I read it. Again and again. I found the place in my city where people came together for this practice, and for a year, I worked up the courage to walk through the doors. I laugh now because I had to give myself permission to stay on the sidelines if that is what needed to be. I live in a body that moves to the beat of whatever music catches its attention! Of course there was no need. I was immediately immersed in the movement. As I played in the Ecstatic Dance practice of 5 Rhythms and Soul Motion and began to move through the stuck places, my body awakened.

I began to understand and experience the sense of walking around ecstatically although I did not connect that with orgasm. It was a state of being incredibly alive and feeling the pleasure centers of my body awakened. All over my body, not just my genitals. The fire that was flickering in my pussy began to smolder and expanded to my hands , my wrists, the bottoms of my feet, my heart, my forehead, my throat, the inside of my mouth ... the sensation of exquisite food as I swallow, ahhhhh, and my sweet, hot belly.

All of these exquisite sensations in my body arising without the focused help of another human, they're just there because I am alive, and

I feel really good! That feeling of aliveness bubbles up from inside, independent of outside stimulation.

I wanted to attach those feelings to a man because I thought that's what I'm supposed to do. I've noticed, though, that whenever I attached that sensation to a man it constricted a little, sometimes a lot, depending on the man. I was mostly too much for them. They would try to fix me. Rein me in. Corral me. And each time that happened the fire in my pussy went into flicker mode. Looking back at it from this perspective, it was me corralling the energy because it is big. It is terrifyingly big and consuming.

And how you do one thing is how you do everything. So my relationship to my orgasm, to my body, to the experience of movement was as chaotic as every other relationship in my life. I've done that with everything and everyone that I have loved!

"Come in close to me."

"No... no... go away, go away!"

Pleasure, ecstasy, orgasm... was no different.

It is ultimately a painful, constrictive way of life, and that way of life took its toll on my body.

A little over midway through 2010, a couple months before I turned 55, I was diagnosed with 14 "MS-like" lesions in my brain, one on my balance center and some rather significant cervical spine compression that required surgery. I had already had surgery on my lower spine the year before, allowing me to continue walking. Now my hands were numb and were not working well, and I got intermittently numb in my genital area ... THAT terrified me more than anything. The thought of no longer being able to give myself pleasure was more than I could bear.

It was very odd, feeling so strongly about losing the ability to pleasure myself because, really? I could lose my mobility. But I had a plan for that. I already knew that I was not going to let that happen. I would not surrender to a wheelchair other than the initial necessity to keep myself post-surgically safe on the uneven path from the parking lot to the stairs leading to my apartment. My neurologist considered me incapacitated (and had the wisdom to keep that to himself until three years later). I was determined to find ways to re-create new neurological connections from brain to limbs. I understood more than most about the neuroplasticity of our brains, and I was fierce in my determination and practice to create new neural pathways.

On the other hand, I wasn't at all sure about my capacity to bring myself to orgasm ever again. I had no idea if my body would ever respond sensually in the way that it had. Touch that used to be pleasurable to my skin was at best irritating, at worst, painful. But I couldn't and wouldn't give up on myself. THAT's how I know that the fire in my pussy doesn't die. Because it didn't when it could have. It heard me. It waited patiently for me to stir it again. It met me. It met me in my bed dances in the middle of the night. I couldn't stand and dance for more than a few minutes, so I would move and stretch in very sensual ways in my bed, in ways that felt good to me and that moved the energy of pleasure through me. I would use my mind to focus it up my spine, down my arms and legs. Sometimes I would bring those sensations to climax. Other times I would let them fade away when they were complete.

I began to practice intentionally stimulating pleasurable sensation by simply moving my body and paying attention to where it started. I also practiced desensitizing the sensation of irritation on my skin. And eventually I touched my clitoris again, slid my fingers into my pussy and tasted its sweetness. The sweetness was still there. The moisture was still there. My vagina still contracted spontaneously in response to my touch.

It is different, however. I can no longer force climax without consequences. Numbness and painful tingling or no feeling at all are among those consequences. Often when I try to force it, I am left with legs that won't settle down as I try to fall asleep. I cannot use it as a release mechanism for whatever needs releasing.

Sometimes, a quiet wail erupts after climax. So much goes into bringing myself to that point, and then it's over! Just like that.

Wailing also because I can feel the fear stuck in my pelvis, and I am so tired of that fear being stuck. And? With every stroke of my clitoris, that fear is loosened. With every stroke, my body is learning a new way to be in the sensation. There are neuro-receptors reconnected between my brain and my pelvis. I am learning a new way to be with my body. My body is learning a new way to be with itself. Something about that soothes me inside.

This is the energy that creates worlds, and it is demanding that I give myself fully into it! How willing am I to surrender into that energy rather than controlling it? How willing am I to surrender into it so that the thing I most desire can express itself? Can I surrender that thing I most desire?

Because this energy that expresses itself as orgasm won't be controlled, and it wants to consume. At the first hint of control, it subsides. My old way of being with it no longer works.

Yes! There is still fire in my 60 year-old pussy. Fire that will not be quenched.

This fire is the expression of life force energy pulsing through me. It is meant to consume me. The thing that scares me more than anything else is the thing I most long for. To be consumed by it. Then and only then, I can be a woman fully intimate with the fire in her own pussy. No matter what! A woman who knows that the fire belongs to her, that it is hers to tend in service to the whole, and that service to the whole starts in service to self. Then and only then, it is truly hers to share as she will.

There is an art to living orgasmically that I am only beginning to understand. It is a force, much like my words, that can be dialed up or down as indicated. In the same way I have asked to know when to speak, and when to listen, I am learning that I can ask it "What do you want? Is this the time to dial up or dial back and just know you're here?" That is the safety mechanism. And that energy can be shifted into ferocity when necessary.

I move my hips ... the pleasure begins in my pelvis and spine. Where I move my hands, sensation starts there and moves through my arms. Wherever the movement initiates, pleasure wants to move through and inform the rest of my body of its presence, teaching the body to receive that level of pleasure. I have been practicing resilience in the face of pain and difficult emotion as I have moved through the trauma and religious deprogramming.

157

Here is the beauty of practicing resilience in the presence of pain. It opens the entire pleasure-pain spectrum. It gives me a skillset, a feeling frame of reference to bring into the practice of pleasure, allowing me to stay in the sensation just a bit longer.

Now I expand that practice into holding pleasure one more notch in this body. And the next and the next and... This beautiful 60 year-old body that has been through everything with me in this life. Surrendering into orgasm is my expression of love to my body. Surrendering into the sensation that rises naturally and expresses as waves of unconstricted pleasure all through my body.

My inner Divine loves to be allowed to hold me and delights in every tiny surrender. That energy lives in every cell of my physical body. Every time I allow it, it bursts forth in sensation from the deep inside out ... I am coming to understand that all I need to do is allow the sensation that is Life Force energy to burst forth from within. It is the surrender of my nervous system to the Inner Divine, to the merging within.

I am home at last.

About the Author
Deborah Penner
www.lovedeepdesign.com

What did you want to be when you were eight years old?

Truthfully? An adult. I had no idea what I wanted to do as an adult. I simply wanted to be one because people listened to what they had to say, and I had a lot to say, and no one listened to children.

If you could give advice to your younger self about your orgasm (or your body), what would it be?

Sweetheart, you are designed to feel immense pleasure. Tune your awareness to that as often as possible. I know it feels impossible at times. Do it anyway. The results will delight you!

If your orgasm had a voice, what would it say to you about the piece you wrote for this book?

Thank you, my love!

SEVENTEEN
HOW TO TURN ME ON
by Mary James

I felt his presence before I saw him.

I was at a wedding reception in Scotland, chatting with my friend, Rachel, about how lucky we were to be two of the chosen ones invited to the wedding. The formal vows had taken place a few hours earlier in an enchanting four hundred year old church. The reception was in a castle.

I'd been in castles before, on tours through the United Kingdom. They were always damp and cold and held the lost dreams of generations of women who felt imprisoned in their own homes. The walls of the castles I'd visited were sturdy and solid and seemed to close in around me as I entered. I always kept an eye out for the nearest exit.

The castle for the wedding reception was different. The land was claimed in the 1100s, and through the years, the walls were built and rebuilt. The final structure, completed in the 1800s, remains today.

Unlike the other castles I'd been in, the walls of this one seduced me. Every room I entered felt better than the last one, as if a feather were being slowly traced across the erogenous zones of my body.

The castle felt safe. Rather than looking for the exit, I wanted to explore every hallway. I was curious to find what lay behind every unopened door.

The minute I felt him, there was also a switch in the music; the pace quickened, and my body passed through a thin veil of consent. I still didn't know what he looked like, but my genitals recognized him and flowed in agreement with what my mind couldn't perceive. A waiter passed by with a tray of champagne.

"Thank you," I said.

"Slàinte," the waiter added.

"To love," Rachel said, and we toasted the possibility that love would exist again for both of us.

I'd been divorced for fifteen years. We had three children and spent several years in therapy, trying to work on our marriage without ever telling the truth. It pushed me too far out of my comfort zone to say what I was feeling, so I stayed quiet rather than risk the consequences of asking for what I wanted.

My husband told the therapist everything that was wrong with me. I sat at the end of the sofa and listened, feeling like I was getting punched with every word. I pulled my shoulders in towards my heart to protect it.

I spent so many years not speaking up that I wasn't even sure who I was anymore. Before children, I had a career that I loved but was quick to give up when I started to give birth to babies instead of ideas. Before marriage, I was self-reliant. I gave that up when I became someone's wife instead of someone's partner. I know I wanted peace in my heart. I know I wanted my children to be content. I know I wanted a husband who valued me. I wasn't sure if it was possible to have all three.

I took an anti-depressant, and instead of looking for answers, I immersed myself in motherhood and took on projects that kept me distracted. My husband took on projects, too. One of them was having sex with our nanny. When I discovered their relationship, I was too numb from the Prozac to care.

We spent more time in therapy so we could save our marriage. I got pregnant again, and we announced to our kids they were going to have a sibling. That was the only change we made. He secretly went back to having sex with our nanny. I miscarried at sixteen weeks. I think the baby knew she was not coming into a family in which she would feel safe.

162

My husband and I grieved in our separate ways. I grieved the loss of the baby with a waiter from Italy. He grieved the loss of the baby by having sex with my best friend. Through it all, I pretended that everything was okay, that I was okay, but really it felt like the walls of those dark castles in the U.K., and I started looking for an exit.

The night of the wedding reception, there was a full moon illuminating everything, including the longing in my heart. When I heard the switch in music from another room, I followed the melody like it was a magnet for my soul, into one of the castle's grand parlors. The ceiling was a sapphire blue. It was all I could see except the backs of the heads of the other wedding guests, more than a hundred of them, in a circle. Their bodies connected through the heat of the moment as they swayed to the sound of the music coming from the center of the circle. And then I saw him.

He was standing on the back of a garnet velvet sofa, balancing himself as he played the saxophone. His fingers rapidly pressed the keys of his instrument, and his breath gave life to each note. Rachel and I turned towards each other at the same time and smiled, and then we pushed our way towards the center of the circle.

His name was William. He was a well-known musician with deep roots in Scottish music. He performed all over the world, but seeing him perform in his home country was like watching him give birth to himself. It was sacred. William was the Jimi Hendrix of saxophone, a man so connected to his instrument that when he played, it was him speaking to you from the source of life that connects us all.

I was mesmerized watching him finger his instrument, bringing the song and the crowd to a peak over and over again. As he played, he made his way across the top of the sofa, over the coffee table, to the side of the circle where Rachel and I stood, and then he leaned into me and asked me to sing. I smiled, but I couldn't find my voice, so he moved on to the next person.

By the time William finished his set, a blanket of euphoria covered the room. We all perspired with the rapture that good music induces as it gives us permission to let our bodies and voices be free. The sound of

William's music faded as he played his way out of the room. I tried to catch up with him but was blocked by the other guests making an exit at the same time.

We got the announcement the wedding cake would be cut in another wing of the castle, so I flowed with the crowd, even though my body was wanting to follow the music.

For the next several hours, the wedding reception roamed from a party in one area of the castle to the next. A band played dance music in the grand ballroom, the wedding cake and desserts were in the solarium, champagne in the garden, Scottish music in the basement bar. I enjoyed the night and celebrated with new friends from all over the world. As the night went on, I looked for William but didn't see him or any of the musicians in his band. He must have left after his set.

I walked the corridors of the castle in wonder, appreciating its walls that were built to embrace and shelter the spirit instead of restraining it. Several places in the castle were engraved with the words *quae sursum volo videre* —" I would see what is heavenly."

Just after midnight, I sneaked outside to stand in the grand gardens under the full moon. I removed my shoes and twirled in my dress, seeing how high I could make the hem fly. It reminded me of the freedom I felt in my body when I was a young girl. Blades of moist grass stuck to my feet as the dress flew higher and higher with only the moon watching me. This is what I wanted in my marriage — the freedom to continue being myself as my partner stood by, enjoying me enjoying myself.

"How's the party?" I stopped dancing to watch a figure coming closer. I knew who it was before I saw his face.

"I like watching you," he said. "I was watching you dance in the ballroom, too."

His words were highlighted by his heavy Scottish burr. I had only heard his voice through his music; now I was hearing him through his words. I smiled.

"You've been here the whole time?" I said.

"Yes," he said. "I didn't have to be anywhere after I played, so I stayed. And I was hoping to see you before I left."

My shoulders pulled back and melted down my spine.

"Do you want to see the rest of the gardens?" he asked, offering me his hand.

I picked up my shoes, took his hand and walked by his side.

For the next several hours we shared stories and then kisses, with the full moon as our chaperone. Before the end of the night, we made plans to see each other the following month when he would be playing near where I lived in the U.S.

A month later, as I prepared for William to arrive at my home, I began to believe the whole thing was too rushed, too much like a fairytale. My mind was cluttered with self-doubt and judgment, but my body was calm and aware of the silent dialogue that began with him in Scotland. I knew I would sleep with him. I wondered if it would be any better, any different than the others.

I'd been with several men since my divorce, and the sex was always the same. They took me hard and fast, and at the end they always asked, "Did you cum?" It was less a question and more a demand. Rather than ask for what I wanted, I played along and smiled and nodded yes. I'd left most of my marriage behind, but I'd not yet remembered that my voice mattered.

I waited outside so he would find the house. He parked his car and walked towards me. Without the castle, the full moon, the gardens and the music, he didn't seem as big as when I last saw him. We stood a few feet from each other and then moved closer until we were almost touching.

"Can I kiss you?" he asked.

His lips caressed my mine until he parted them with gentle nudges of his tongue. My mind quieted as currents of energy animated my body. It all felt perfect, and then an hour later it did not.

"Let's keep this private," he said in his thick accent, or at least that's what I thought he said. We'd been catching up over a cup of tea inside my house and already discussing when we could see each other again.

What I heard was, *I don't value you.* I should have asked him what he meant, but I kept quiet.

I slouched when he started to kiss me again. The previous spark in his lips was gone, or maybe it was the spark in mine. I didn't feel anything. *Don't withdraw*, I pleaded with myself. *You can let him go, but don't let yourself go. Don't disappear like you did in your marriage.*

I allowed the kiss to continue a few minutes longer, trying to turn myself back on.

Nothing.

His hands started playing me, fingering me like I was the keys on his saxophone. *Too fast*, I thought but still stayed quiet. My body tightened from my lack of communication.

He sensed the change, like a song being played in the wrong key. He pulled away enough to give me space, but not enough to let me go.

"Everything okay?" he asked.

Tears filled my eyes. Don't do this. Please don't cry. Don't reveal yourself.

And then I heard a sound come through my mouth. It was shaking a little, but it was still forming words. It was my voice.

"Earlier when you said you wanted to keep me a secret, it made me feel like you didn't value being with me. I am not someone to hide."

He looked at me with tender eyes. I continued.

"I really enjoyed our time together in Scotland, and I'm happy we're seeing each other again, but I don't want to be with another man who doesn't appreciate me, whether it's for one date or a lifetime."

My voice stopped shaking even as the words and tears kept flowing.

He kept listening until I said everything I needed to say to him, to past lovers, to past boyfriends, to my ex-husband.

Two things surprised me by the time I finished talking. He was still listening, and I was turned on. It never occurred to me that every time in the past when I didn't speak up, I was also shutting down the energy to my genitals. I felt the wetness through my panties and the longing in my body, and the odd thing was, it wasn't for him. It was a response to finally valuing myself and speaking up. I was turned on by speaking my truth, even if it made me uncomfortable.

I started to pull away because I thought he would want to, as well. It seemed like too much information to offer a new man in my life. He pulled me closer, and I rested my head on his chest. We lay together for a long time listening to the silence between us.

"Why are you still here?" I asked. "Don't you think I sounded a little crazy with everything I just told you?"

"I think that somewhere in your life, you must have been hurt by a man or men, and if you can get it out, you'll be okay.

Are you okay now?"

"I'm okay," I said, and for the first time in my life, it really felt like the truth.

About the Author
Mary Jane

What did you want to be when you were eight years old?

I wanted to be a writer. I wrote poems first, then short stories.

If you could give advice to your younger self about your orgasm (or your body), what would it be?

I wish I had asked more questions about my body instead of feeling scared and uncomfortable in my skin. I was a curious child, and I asked a lot of questions and explored, except when it came to my body. I'm sure the early abuse kept me from being curious.

If your orgasm had a voice, what would it say to you about the piece you wrote for this book?

I'm glad that you slowed down and finally spoke up.

EIGHTEEN

WHAT MY ORGASM WANTS TO TELL YOU

by Betsy Blankenbaker

After releasing *Autobiography of an Orgasm* in 2014, I started receiving letters and messages from women and several men who read the book and were affected by my choice to tell such a vulnerable story.

"Thank you for speaking up."

"This is a courageous book."

"You've shown me how to stop judging myself and appreciate myself instead."

"I was meant to read your book. I see myself in your story and now I see that I can heal too."

"Thank you for your book. I think it might help me start living."

"Your book made me excited about exploring sex again instead of being ashamed."

"You are changing the world and how we think about sex."

What is the story of your orgasm? Do you have a story you would like to be considered for the next volume of *Autobiographies of Our Orgasms*? This isn't *Fifty Shades of Grey*. It's women and men telling true stories from their sensual paths. Ideally, you will choose to write and publish under your name, but it you aren't ready to speak up with your name attached, you can publish under a pseudonym.

To be considered for the book, please submit your story of up to 4,000 words to: aoaothebook@gmail.com.

www.betsyblankenbaker.com
Betsy can be contacted at aoaothebook@gmail.com
or you can 'Follow' her on Facebook: Betsy Blankenbaker

ACKNOWLEDGEMENTS

Thank you to all the writers featured in this book for writing about events in their lives, especially the moments that felt too private to tell but that you wrote down anyway. Through your stories, we remember that our lives matter and that love is always present, even in the times when we felt the most alone, abandoned or betrayed. Your stories show us how you danced the path back to yourselves and remind us that we can find our way home, too.

Thank you to Paul Yinger for the beautiful cover designs for this book. Thank you for making my Os look so good!

Thank you to my friend, novelist and writing teacher Dan Wakefield, for standing for my orgasm, my books and my films and for adding his words to the cover of the book.

Thank you to Dr. Liz Orchard for being a valued expert on women's bodies and wellness. Thank you for adding your words to the Forward of this book.

Thank you to the communities of Ubud, Bali and Byron Bay, Australia where I completed the final work on this collection.

Thank you to my friend Rochelle Schieck for creating Qoya (loveqoya.com) so I could remember my body and life as sacred.

Thank you to my friend Sao for reminding me that writing is how my soul breathes.

Thank you to my fantastic copy editor (and sometimes cheerleader), Amanda Coffin.

Thank you to the Smith sisters for listening to some of these stories over dinners. Thank you to Dee for always listening.

Thank you to my children Sam, Lucy, Willie and Charlie for being so understanding and supportive when I chose to write about orgasm.

Made in the USA
Charleston, SC
24 March 2016